Mnemonics
and Study Tips
for Medical Students

D1421621

Mnemonics and Study Tips
for Medical Students

Two Zebras Borrowed My Car

Third Edition

Khalid Khan BSc(Pharmacy) MRPharmS MBBS(London) MRCGP DRCOG DFFP DCH DCM(Beijing), GP Principal, Surrey, UK

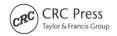

CRC Press
Taylor & Francis Group

CRC Press
Taylor & Francis Group
6000 Broken Sound Parkway NW, Suite 300
Boca Raton, FL 33487-2742

© 2016 by Khalid Khan
CRC Press is an imprint of Taylor & Francis Group, an Informa business

No claim to original U.S. Government works

Printed in Great Britain by Ashford Colour Press Ltd
Version Date: 20160505

International Standard Book Number-13: 978-1-4987-3938-2 (Paperback)

Library of Congress Cataloging-in-Publication Data

Names: Khan, Khalid, Dr., author.
Title: Mnemonics and study tips for medical students / Khalid Khan.
Description: Third edition. | Boca Raton : Taylor & Francis, 2016. | Includes
bibliographical references and index.
Identifiers: LCCN 2016006331 | ISBN 9781498739382 (paperback : alk. paper)
Subjects: | MESH: Medicine | Association Learning | Examination Questions
Classification: LCC R737 | NLM WB 18.2 | DDC 610.76--dc23
LC record available at http://lccn.loc.gov/2016006331

Visit the Taylor & Francis Web site at
http://www.taylorandfrancis.com

and the CRC Press Web site at
http://www.crcpress.com

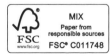

mnemonic /nemonik. L mnemonicus f. Gk mnemonikos
derives from Mnemosyne, ancient Greek goddess. A memory aid
or pertaining to aiding the memory. Often considered to be a code,
device, acronym or formula to facilitate memory or understanding.
The term is used here in its broadest possible sense.

Please return this book to:

CONTENTS

PREFACE: FREQUENTLY ASKED QUESTIONS

For the insatiably curious...

Q. So what exactly is a mnemonic?

The name comes from the Greek goddess of memory, Mnemosyne, the mother of the muses and means 'remembrance'. A mnemonic is essentially any type of memory aid. The term is used here in the broadest possible sense, to include any tool or device that makes learning easier (not just codes or anagrams).

Q. Will learning somebody else's mnemonic help me?

Given that they may have been used for generations, it's just possible that they will actually help. You'll remember your own mnemonics best because they'll be derived from the way your own mind works and will draw on your own particular strengths – hence some tips in Section III on making our own. You can still benefit from somebody else's knowledge or ideas – that's why you are at university in the first place!

Q. Well, I know people who've never used a mnemonic in the whole of their medical career.

Well think of, for example, the APGAR score – it is actually a mnemonic, and your first-aid treatment of sprains might be a bit rusty too (see PRICE). There's ROY G BIV for the colours of the spectrum (or 'Richard of York Gave Battle In Vain'), and 'Every Good Boy Deserves Football' for music notes. Another example is the modified Glasgow criteria for predicting severity of pancreatitis PANCREAS in which P stands for PaO2 (< 8 kPa); A for age (> 55); N for neutrophils ≠; C for calcium (< 2 mM); R for renal urea (> 16 mM); E for enzymes (LDH, lactate dehydrogenase > 6000 IU/L; AST, aspartate aminotransferase > 200 IU/L); A for albumin ↓; and S for sugar > 10 mM).

Q. Why make revising medicine funny?

Humour is useful as a learning tool – just because something is serious doesn't mean it has to be miserable. Besides, humour coaxes your mind into producing more 'feel good' neurotransmitters and hormones such as oxytocin, enhancing the learning experience – you are more likely to be interested in something you enjoy. In fact, humour has been used for centuries by doctors who are often exposed daily to the grimmest realities and horrors of human fragility. Humour is a coping mechanism and a release mechanism; it helps you keep your sanity and allows you to give your best to your patients.

When a patient first sees you, they have no idea what you have seen or done just before their meeting with you – and neither should they – and they will still expect you to greet them warmly, hopefully with a smile, and ideally with a reassuring twinkle in your eye. If you feel good, so will they – just try looking totally miserable the next time you see a new patient and see how well that goes! Peter Ustinov once said that comedy is simply a funny way of being serious.

Q. So things like interest and humour may help more than mnemonics?

Exactly.

Q. The effort of learning these acronyms in the first place makes mnemonics pointless. What on earth is SALFOPSM for instance?

I agree. Not all of this type of mnemonic is easy or useful. I have attempted to limit these. They do become more useful if the first two letters are used, or if a rhyming word or phonetically similar letter is used – and you will notice plenty of these in this book. SALFOPSM is one mnemonic where you have to use a lot of effort to learn what it means and, although it is used by many students, I think it is quite difficult.

For the more curious among you, the branches of the external carotid artery are given by SALFOPSM thus: S for superior thyroid; A for ascending pharyngeal; L for lingual; F for facial; O for occipital; P for posterior auricular; S for superior temporal; M for maxillary. And for the internal carotid you can use OPCAM – but I'll let you work that out for yourself.

Q. I've read about short-term and long-term memory. Do memory aids have something to do with this?

Yes. Generally most information enters your 'short-term' memory first and, then, by an unknown physiological process is stored permanently as a 'long-term' memory. All memory aids and systems work by linking your new information to an already-existing piece of memory – something that you already know. In this process of association, the new knowledge gets a 'piggy-back' on the long-term memory, meaning you can assimilate the required knowledge quicker because your neurons have to make fewer new physiological changes (otherwise your brain would be making neuronal connections in a long-winded, tedious and random way).

Q. So association is the basis of an efficient memory?

Essentially, yes.

Q. And you say that physiological changes actually happen when memories are made?

Yes. The evidence for this has been accumulating for quite some time. One example is illustrated by the brains of London taxi-drivers. Researchers at University College London scanned the brains of 16 cabbies and found that the hippocampus enlarges after they underwent 'knowledge' training.

Q. What about dual-hemisphere brain-learning techniques?

Well, the best way to learn is to use both hemispheres of the brain. This bilateral learning is coaxed and encouraged by the use of memory aids. It is inherent in the very nature of mnemonics. A good mnemonic will make use of the analytical and critical areas of your brain as well as the visual and creative parts. You will notice that the more sensory modalities you use (like smell, touch and sight) the easier it is to remember things. The more extreme the sensory input, the more likely you are to remember it – the more vivid the picture, the stronger the smell, the more energetic the associated emotions, the stronger the connotations, the more powerful the memory will be, and the more likely it is to be coded into long-term physiological memory.

Q. I find that the mnemonics disappear after a while, because I don't need them anymore… because I just know.

Exactly! This happens when the facts become part of your long-term memory – you need mnemonic it no more – because you know more!

Q. All the mnemonics I have heard are rude.

They don't have to be rude or offensive to be useful – although sometimes this helps the associative process. Too many similar phrases defeat the object of the exercise, so I have not used many here. Although the rude ones can be very popular, they have their limitations as learning tools. (Some students complain that they are not offensive enough!)

Q. But don't they just offend half the students while making the other half giggle?

Actually the rudest, most offensive and explicit mnemonics I know about were supplied almost entirely by female medical students. Most of these are unpublishable, so I haven't included them here. Anyway, some don't make particularly good memory aids, especially because it can be confusing trying to remember who does what to whom!

Q. What about mistakes?

I quote Aeschylus (the ancient Greek playwright) who said: 'The wisest of the wise may err.' So apologies in advance – just in case. Anyway, these mnemonics do not replace your regular course notes, and they do not replace any existing or past guidelines or accepted clinical practices. They are simply to help with your revision. They do not replace clinical judgement or methodology, nor are they a substitute for any part of your training. But please do send your comments and/or point out any of the 'deliberate' mistakes! You can email me at kk2@doctors.org.uk.

Q. Should I be making notes in the margin?

It will help you to learn. I have even left some space for your own scribbles. Jotting and doodling involve more areas of your brain, reinforcing the memories and crystallizing those thoughts in your mind. The process of using your hands in addition to both brain hemispheres contributes to whole-brain learning – and it will make you a better learner.

Q. So as I read and learn, this book – funny, yet serious – will show me techniques for association and how to use humour to evoke interest and stimulate my neurological memory to its fullest potential, while also giving me the tools to devise my own mnemonics and study techniques, so maximizing the efficiency of my revision time?

Exactly! Well said!

Q. And there are no rules in mnemonics, except to do what works?

Precisely!

KK, 2016

WHY *THIS* BOOK IS SO GOOD!

Congratulations! You are a student of one of the most exciting undergraduate courses in the world. Time and knowledge are precious; you will be challenged in countless directions, with constant syllabus changes, and you will be expected to assimilate a colossal amount of raw knowledge. Therefore, you need to manage your time and energies efficiently. Herein lies some assistance.

This compilation of medical mnemonics places the emphasis on user-friendliness. Those that are quickest to assimilate are given priority, so many popular, old favourites are included, and there is guidance on how to study efficiently and create your own memory aids. You will remember many of these forever, and with minimal effort. Remember, this book will be there for you all the way from freshers to graduation and beyond…

Einstein said that if there is an easier way – find it! There are some easier ways in this magical volume. Go find 'em!

Welcome to the new edition

Welcome to the third edition of the UK's first ever book of contextualized mnemonics.

It was great news when the publishers, after consultation with student reviewers, requested a new edition. This is at a time when thousands of mnemonics are available online, so we were delighted to discover that so many of you find this quirky and unique publication so helpful. As before, you still love the 'swot' boxes, limericks, study tips, pegs and that shameless infusion of fun oozing from cover to cover. We have also added a new feature of 'Jot Boxes' to this edition to encourage you to add your own notes and create your own mnemonics as you go.

This text was never intended to be just a list of anagrams or a comprehensive textbook of medicine. It is designed to be portable, affordable and friendly, to be a veritable antidote to the stress and despair so prevalent around exam time, and to provide you with encouragement through the oodles of hope and good feelings crammed into every word on every page.

The challenge has always been to keep the book small and the costs down. While this little text is slowly morphing into something of a study guide in addition to the mnemonics, my original mission still stands – go make your learning fast, fun and magical at every opportunity.

KK, 2016

kk2@doctors.org.uk

ACKNOWLEDGEMENTS

This publication would not have been possible without the help, cooperation and encouragement of hundreds of students from various medical schools and colleges over many years. Although many of the innovators of mnemonics over the centuries will remain anonymous (and therefore cannot be specifically credited here), I wish in particular to give my thanks to following people:

Aamir Zafar
Aidan Mowbray
Amer Shoaib
Andrew Eldridge
Atique Imam
Caroline Hallett
Chris Menzies
Debbie Rogers
Dia Karanough
Dush Mital
Elizabeth Picton
Fatima Zafar
Georgina Bentliffe
Gwen Andradi
Hammad Malik
Harvey Chant
Helen Marsden
John Morlese
Kate Ward
Kevin Chua
Khalid Hassan
'Kuz'
Leigh Urwin
Mahmooda Qureshi

Majeed Musalam
Maryam Zafar
Matt Jones
Megan Morris
Milan Radia
Nazneen Ala
Neil Bhatia
Nicola Carter
Paul Kennedy
Paul McCoubrie
Paul Roome
Puja Patel
Quinn Scobies
Raj Bhargava
'Rats'
Raza Toosey
Rebekah Garnham
Rob Ward
Dr Robert Clarke ('The Barnet course')
Sana Haroon
Shahid Khan
Sheetle Shah
Sophie Shaw
Stuart McCorkel

Thanks also to the General Management Committee of the St George's Hospital Medical School Club (SGUL Students Union), and my extra special thanks go to Professor Aftab Ala of The Royal Surrey County Hospital.

Every effort has been made to trace the original sources and copyright holders and to cite them in this book, but in this large compilation we recognize this has not always been possible. Those we have not included citations for are either anonymous, or no one has declared ownership of them! To this end, any individual who claims copyright for any mnemonic in this book should contact the publisher, so that an acknowledgement may be included in future editions.

Please note that all characters in this book are entirely fictional and do not in any way relate to real persons, alive or dead. The only exceptions are those people whose sayings or quotes I have given acknowledgement or credit to.

BASIC MEDICAL SCIENCES

ANATOMY

Anatomy is destiny

Sigmund Freud

Our adventure begins with anatomy – where most students of medicine first come across mnemonics. Try this short quiz before you start reading.

PRE-QUIZ

1 Can you name the carpal bones?
2 What is the nerve supply to the diaphragm?
3 What are the posterior relations of the kidney?
4 Which palmar interossei abduct?
5 Which structures pass through the lesser sciatic foramen?
6 Which pain fibres carry crude touch sensations?
7 Which modalities are carried in the dorsal columns?
8 How many dermatomes do you know?

1.1 THE UPPER LIMB

Carpal bones

The eight small bones in the wrist are arranged in two rows of four. Imagine the proximal row of the wrist (Latin = *carpus*), from lateral to medial. You will see the scaphoid, lunate, triquetral and pisiform. Then visualize the distal row, going the other way from medial to lateral: you will see the hamate, capitate, trapezoid, trapezium. Here is an old favourite for remembering their sequence.

Sue Likes Terry's Pens – Her Cap's Too Tight

Sue	**S**caphoid	
Likes	**L**unate	PROXIMAL ROW
Terry's	**T**riquetral	
Pens	**P**isiform	
Her	**H**amate	
Cap's	**C**apitate	DISTAL ROW
Too	**T**rapezoid	
Tight	**T**rapezium	

Variations include changing the people's names or using alternatives to 'pen' and 'cap', but they are all too rude to print here! If this is still too difficult for you to remember, try this elegant version in which both rows of carpal bones go from lateral to medial.

Some Lovers Try Positions That They Cannot Handle

Some	**S**caphoid	
Lovers	**L**unate	PROXIMAL ROW
Try	**T**riquetral	
Positions	**P**isiform	
That	**T**rapezium	
They	**T**rapezoid	DISTAL ROW
Cannot	**C**apitate	
Handle	**H**amate	

Locate on your own wrist to see which bone you can most easily remember. This action will help to reinforce the memory associations in your brain.

SWOT BOX

Now is a good time to remind you that the scaphoid (in the snuffbox) is the most commonly shattered bone in the wrist (and sometimes is not seen on X-ray for some 2 weeks or so).

Cubital fossa

Some students visualize Madeline Brown's Big Red Pustule to remember features of the cubital fossa. From medial to lateral, embedded in fat, you will find the median nerve, brachial artery, biceps tendon, radial nerve and posterior interosseous nerve.

Madeline Brown's Big Red Pustule

Madeline	**M**edian nerve
Brown's	**B**rachial artery
Big	**B**iceps tendon
Red	**R**adial nerve
Pustule	**P**osterior interosseous nerve

Alternatives

Mr Brown Bites Rabbits Posteriorly

Madeline Brown's Big Radiology Posting

Madeline Brown's Big Red Pussy

Note that these characters are purely fictitious and are not based on anybody who ever existed. Mr Brown's rabbit gave the author verbal permission.

Interossei muscles of the hand

There are four palmar and four dorsal interossei. They all have ulnar nerve innervation. Think of PAD and DAB to help you remember what they do.[1]

PAD and DAB

PAD	**P**almar interossei **AD**duct
DAB	**D**orsal interossei **AB**duct

Latissimus dorsi

This is an old, anonymous and easy way of remembering that the latissimus dorsi muscle is attached to the humerus, on the floor of the bicipital groove, with the tendon between the attachments of the pectoralis major and teres major.

1 From Moore KL (1985) *Clinical Orientated Anatomy*, 2nd edn. Philadelphia: Williams & Wilkins.

Lady Doris Between Two Majors

Lady Doris	latissimus dorsi
(between)	(between)
Two **Majors**	pectoralis **major** and teres **major**

Rotator cuff

To remember the rotator cuff, think of the word 'sits'. This describes how the attachments of the rotator cuff muscles to the humerus.

SItS[2]

S	**S**upraspinatus
I	**I**nfraspinatus
t	**t**eres minor
S	**S**ubscapularis

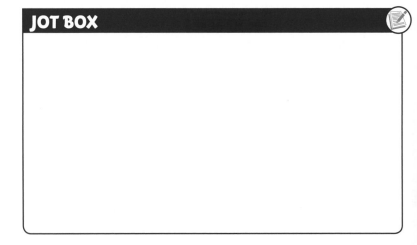

Supraspinatus
Infraspinatus
teres minor (hence little 't')
Subscapularis

JOT BOX

---

2 An original from Atique Imam FRCS, 1987.

1.2 THE THORAX

Costal groove

The well-known sequence of important structures in the costal groove at the inferior border of the rib, going inferiorly, are the vein, artery and nerve.

VAN

V	**V**ein
A	**A**rtery
N	**N**erve

This is how these structures lie alongside a rib.

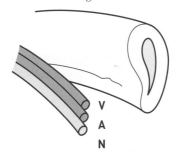

Diaphragm

This simple rhyming verse will always remind you that the nerve supply to the diaphragm is via the third, fourth and fifth cervical nerve roots.

C 3, 4 and 5
Keep the diaphragm alive!

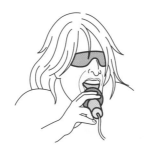

Lingual nerve

The lingual nerve takes a swerve
around the hyoglossus
Said Wharton's duct 'Well I'll be f****d
The bugger's double-crossed us!'

Several doctors and students contributed this one over the years so presumably it has been used a lot. Even though it has been around for decades, the original source has not been found.

Phrenic nerve

Here is the simple use of a pattern to make an association.

The **ph**renic nerve
is in **ph**ront of the trachea

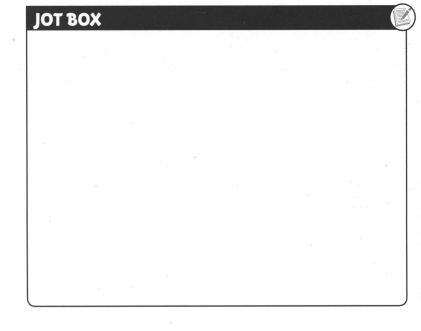

JOT BOX

1.3 THE ABDOMEN AND PELVIS

Anal and urethral sphincters

You can remember that the second, third and fourth sacral nerve roots supply these sphincters from this simple rhyme.

S 2, 3 and 4
Keep the pee off the floor!

NAUGHTY BIT

Some authorities use a suitably 'shitty' word to describe the function of the anal sphincter. Choose whatever term you find most... err... convenient.

The kidney

The posterior relations of the kidney are similar on both sides of the body (the anterior relations are different).

SWOT BOX

There is one artery – the subcostal. Two bones – the eleventh and twelfth ribs – are deep to the diaphragm. Three nerves – the subcostal, iliohypogastric and ilioinguinal – descend diagonally. Posteriorly, the superior pole of the kidney is related to four muscles – the diaphragm, the quadratus lumborum (more inferiorly), the psoas major (medially) and the transversus abdominis (laterally).

Try to remember this number sequence '1, 2, 3, 4' and this phrase 'all boys need muscle'. Now consider the following:

1-2-3-4 All Boys Need Muscle

1	**A**ll	**A**rtery
2	**B**oys	**B**ones
3	**N**eed	**N**erves
4	**M**uscle	**M**uscle

Alternative

A cheeky alternative for readers who are a lost cause is:

Altered **B**oys **N**ever **M**asturbate

(and derivatives thereof).

Renal arteries

To remember the branches of the renal arteries, cross your hands in front of you, at the wrist, as shown in the picture. The thumb represents the single posterior segment branch of the renal artery and the four fingers represent the four main anterior segmental arteries.[3]

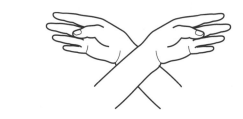

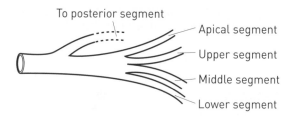

To posterior segment

Apical segment

Upper segment

Middle segment

Lower segment

Thumb	Posterior segment branch
2nd Finger	Apical segment branch
3rd Finger	Upper segment branch
4th Finger	Middle segment branch
5th Finger	Lower segment branch

3 From Blandy J (1988) *Lecture Notes in Urology*, 4th edn. Oxford: Blackwell.

The spleen

A useful description of the spleen (albeit in imperial measures!) is that it is 1 by 3 by 5 inches in size, it weighs 7 ounces, and it lies obliquely between the ninth and eleventh ribs. To be able to regurgitate all this information, seamlessly, simply remember the number sequence.

1-3-5-7-9-11

1	**1** inch
3	**3** inches
5	**5** inches
7	**7** ounces
9	**9**th rib
11	**11**th rib

Superior mesenteric artery

The superior mesenteric artery is one of those structures that arises at the level of the transpyloric plane and L1. It ends by anastamosing with one of its own branches – the ileocolic.

MRI[4]

M	**M**id-colic artery
R	**R**ight colic artery
I	**I**leocolic artery

JOT BOX

4 Attributed to Faisal Raza at University of East Anglia Medical School.

1.4 THE LOWER LIMB

Ankle joint tendons

Inferior to the medial malleolus are the tendons of the tibialis posterior, flexor digitorum longus, posterior tibial artery, posterior tibial nerve and flexor hallucis longus.

Tom, Dick And Harry

Tom	**T**ibialis posterior
Dick	Flexor **d**igitorum longus
And	Posterior tibial **a**rtery and posterior tibial **n**erve
Harry	Flexor **h**allucis longus

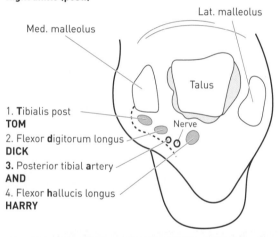

Right ankle (post.)

Lat. malleolus

Med. malleolus

Talus

1. **T**ibialis post
TOM

Nerve

2. Flexor **d**igitorum longus
DICK

3. Posterior tibial **a**rtery
AND

4. Flexor **h**allucis longus
HARRY

SWOT BOX

The ankle is the most frequently injured major joint in the body. Its nerves are the tibial and deep peroneal. The lateral ligament, which is the most frequently damaged, attaches the lateral malleolus to the talus calcaneus. Arterial supply to the joint is via the tibial arteries (peroneal, anterior and posterior).

The femoral triangle

The femoral triangle can be found as a depression inferior to the inguinal ligament (the base of the femoral triangle). Medially is the adductor longus and laterally is the sartorius (this is more obvious if the thigh is flexed, abducted and laterally rotated).

It is handy when you need to take blood via a femoral 'stab' or perform left cardiac angiographies to think of the word NAVY – but you do need to know where your Y-fronts are for this to work!

NAVY

N	**N**erve
A	**A**rtery
V	**V**ein
Y	**Y**-fronts

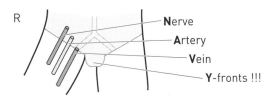

R

Nerve
Artery
Vein
Y-fronts !!!

And going medial to lateral, the floor of the triangle consists of the pectineus, iliacus, and psoas major – giving you PIMP.

PIMP

P	**P**ectineus
I	**I**liacus
MP	**P**soas **m**ajor

SWOT BOX

Femoral hernias arise just inferolateral to the pubic tubercle, below the inguinal ligament, medial to the femoral vein. They are more common in women owing to their wider pelvis.

Lesser sciatic foramen

This mnemonic will remind you that the nerve to the obturator internus, and its tendon and pudendal nerve and pudendal vessels pass through the lesser sciatic foramen.

No Internals Tonight, Padre

No Internals	**N**erve to **o**bturator **i**nternus
Tonight	**T**endon
Padre	**P**udendal nerve/vessels

The patella – Is it a left one or a right one?

Place the patella with the posterior surface on the table in front of you with the inferior border (pointy corner) pointing away from you (distally). How it comes to rest on the table will show you whether it is from a left or a right knee.

Resting on its **right** side	From a **right** knee
Resting on its **left** side	From a **left** knee

The pelvis – Golly, is it male or female?

Just look at the shape of the greater sciatic notch to find out which is which.

Lucy (female)	**L**-shaped sciatic notch
Johnnie (male)	**J**-shaped sciatic notch

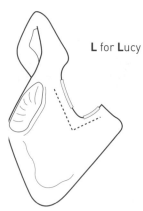

L for **L**ucy

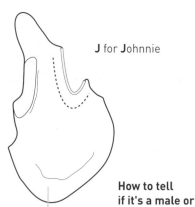

J for **J**ohnnie

Inominate bone

How to tell if it's a male or female pelvis

Sartorius and gracilis muscles

This elegant memory aid has long been used to remind us that the sartorius and gracilis are attached to the medial surface of the tibia just before (i.e. anteriorly) to the semitendinosus.

Say Grace Before Tea

Say	**S**artorius
Grace	**g**racilis
Before	**Before**

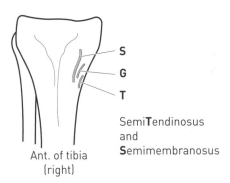

S
G
T

Semi**T**endinosus
and
Semimembranosus

Ant. of tibia
(right)

Tea	Semi**T**endinosus

Supine or prone?

Any difficulty with these tricky terms is easily resolved with:

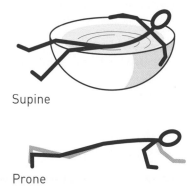

Supine

Prone

Supine – like a bowl of **soup**
Prone – like doing **pr**ess-ups

The thigh

There are five **adductor muscles** of the thigh – the pectineus, gracilis, adductor longus, adductor brevis and adductor magnus. These muscles are all supplied by the obturator nerve, except for the pectineus (femoral nerve). Part of the adductor magnus is also supplied by the sciatic nerve. They generally originate from the pubis. As well as adducting, they are important in fixating the hip joint and for normal gait. You will remember them with the help of this phrase.

Observe Three Ducks Pecking Grass

Observe	**O**bturator
Three Ducks	three A**ddu**ctors
Pecking	**P**ectineus
Grass	**G**racilis

SWOT BOX

The gracilis (and its nerves and vessels) may be used surgically to repair damaged muscle. It is a relatively weak muscle and its loss has a minimal effect on leg adduction. Incidentally, tears or strains of the adductor muscles are common in fast bowlers (cricket) while ossification of the adductor longus can occur in horse riders.

Now consider the **posterior compartments** of the thigh. In ancient times these muscles (the hamstrings) were slashed in order to bring down enemy horses, and even to prevent prisoners from running away![5] On a lighter note, here comes Swotty Samantha – note, she is a purely fictitious character.

Big Fat Swotty Samantha Ate My Hamster's Pens

Big Fat	**B**iceps **f**emoris
Swo**tt**y	**S**emi**t**endinous
Sam**a**ntha	**S**emi**m**embranous
Ate **M**y	**A**dductor **m**agnus
Hamster's Pens	**Hamst**ring **p**ortion

5 From Moore KL (1985) *Clinical Orientated Anatomy*, 2nd edn. Philadelphia: Williams & Wilkins.

1.5 THE HEAD AND NECK

Carotid sheath

This is a portion of tubular cervical fascia enclosing the vagus nerve, carotid artery and internal jugular vein. AJAX is a quick way to remember what is in it.

AJAX

A	**A**rtery number 1 (the common carotid)
J	**J**ugular vein
A	**A**rtery number 2 (the internal carotid)
X	**X**th cranial nerve (the vagus)

NAVY works as a useful formula too.

NAVY

N	**N**erve (the vagus)
A	**A**rteries (the common and internal carotids)
V	**V**ein (the internal jugular)
Y	**Y**-shape (rough shape made by the two terminal branches of the common carotid artery)

SWOT BOX

The carotid sheath extends from the base of the skull to the thorax. If the large vessels mentioned here are moved during surgery, the vagus nerve will be moved with them.

Circle of Willis

Have you met Willis the spider? Students often find it helpful to visualize a spider like this one, with a face, eight legs... and a Willis.[6]

He has a face   Eight legs   And a Willis...!

6 Derived from a concept in Goldberg S (2007) *Clinical Anatomy Made Ridiculously Simple*. MedMaster.

And when you put them all together, it suddenly makes sense.

'Willis the spider'

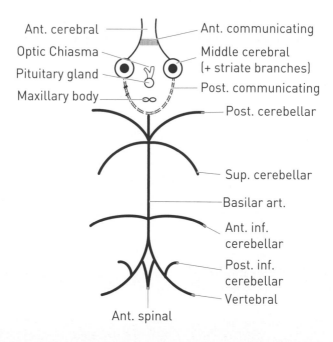

Ant. cerebral — Ant. communicating
Optic Chiasma — Middle cerebral (+ striate branches)
Pituitary gland — Post. communicating
Maxillary body — Post. cerebellar
Sup. cerebellar
Basilar art.
Ant. inf. cerebellar
Post. inf. cerebellar
Vertebral
Ant. spinal

Don't forget that old exam favourite – the pontine branches.

SWOT BOX

The anterior cerebral arteries are involved in 30% of subarachnoid haemorrhages; the middle and posterior cerebral arteries each account for 25%.

JOT BOX

Cranial fossa foramens

There are four middle cranial fossa openings, one of which is the **superior orbital fissure**.

The structures passing through the superior orbital fissure are the lacrimal nerve, frontal nerve, trochlear nerve, the superior division of cranial nerve III, oculomotor nerve (to superior oblique), nasociliary nerve, the inferior division of cranial nerve III and the abducens nerve (VI). A very old, oft-quoted mnemonic is:

Lazy French Tarts Sprawl Naked In Anticipation

Lazy	**La**crimal
French	**F**rontal
Tarts	**T**rochlear
Sprawl	**S**uperior division of III (nerve to superior oblique) – oculomotor
Naked	**N**asociliary
In	**In**ferior division of III
Anticipation	**A**bducens

SWOT BOX

The **superior orbital fissure** lies between the lateral wall and the roof of the orbit. It allows structures to communicate with the middle cranial fossa. A penetrating injury to the eye can therefore enter the middle cranial fossa and the frontal lobe of the brain. The superior orbital fissure meets the inferior orbital fissure at the apex of the orbit.

The other three main openings of the middle cranial fossa are the **foramen rotundum**, **ovale** and **spinosum**; the first two are in the greater wing of the sphenoid and the third (as its name suggests) is near the spine of the sphenoid.

ROS

R	Foramen **R**otundum
O	Foramen **O**vale
S	Foramen **S**pinosum

External carotid artery

I don't personally feel that this anonymous mnemonic is especially good, but it is undoubtedly favoured by some students.

SALFOPSM

S	**S**uperior thyroid
A	**A**scending pharyngeal
L	**L**ingual
F	**F**acial
O	**O**ccipital
P	**P**osterior auricular
S	**S**uperior temporal
M	**M**axillary

How about creating your own (better) memory jogger for these structures?

Foramen magnum

The important structures passing through the foramen magnum are easily remembered by this phrase – as long as you say it with a German accent! Helpful in a clinch (but no apologies if it isn't)!

Limp Sympathetic Men *Vear* Corduroy Accessories

Limp	Meningeal **lymp**hatics
Sympathetic	**Sympathetic** plexus (on the vertebral arteries)
Men	**Men**inges
Vear	**Ve**rtebral **ar**teries (+ spinal branches)
Corduroy	Spinal **Cord**
Accessories	**Accessory** nerves

Foramens of Luschka and Magendie

The roof of the fourth ventricle has three foramens – the medial foramen of Magendie and two foramens of Luschka. The cerebrospinal fluid leaves via these openings into the subarachnoid space. This is how to remember the location of these foramens.[7]

Magendie	**M**edial
Luschka	**L**ateral

7 From Gertz SD, Gaithersburg MD (1996) *Liebman's Neuroanatomy Made Easy and Understandable*, 3rd edn. Aspen Publishers.

Layers of the scalp

This is a very popular mnemonic judging by the number of texts it is quoted in – and justifiably so.

SCALP

S	**S**kin
C	**C**onnective tissue
A	**A**poneurosis
L	**L**oose connective tissue
P	**P**eriosteum

Maxillary nerve

There is also a neat way to remind yourself that the maxillary nerve exits the skull via the foramen rotundum and the mandibular nerve via the foramen ovale.

Max Returns Mandy's Ovum...

MAX	**MAX**illary nerve
Returns	foramen **R**otundum
MANDy's	**MAND**ibular nerve
OVum	foramen **OV**ale

You can add another phrase to this to remind you that the important middle meningeal artery passes through the foramen spinosum, giving you 'Max Returns Mandy's Ovum… May Marry Spinster'.

May Marry Spinster

May **MAR**ry	**M**iddle **M**eningeal **AR**tery
SPINster	foramen **SPIN**osum

JOT BOX

Parasympathetic ganglia

The four parasympathetic ganglia are the ciliary, otic, pterygopalatine and sub-mandibular. Here is a simple mnemonic to remember them.

COPS

C	**C**iliary
O	**O**tic
P	**P**terygopalatine
S	**S**ubmandibular

If this is far too boring (and you are not the politically correct type), then perhaps this modified but rather unflattering phrase of sound-likes and initial letters will be more memorable to you.

Silly Old People Stay Mouldy

Silly	**Cili**ary
Old	**O**ptic
People	**P**terygopalatine
Stay **M**ouldy	**S**ub**M**andibular

SWOT BOX

The ciliary ganglion is in the posterior orbit. The oculomotor nerve (III) goes here too. Postganglionic fibres supply the ciliary muscle and pupils. The hypoglossal (IX) nerve supplies the otic ganglion and connects to the parotid gland, causing salivation. The pterygopalatine (or sphenopalatine) ganglion lies in its own fossa; nerve fibres come from the facial nerve (VII), supplying the lacrimal, nasal and palatine glands. The submandibular ganglion has fibres from the facial nerve (VII); it supplies the sublingual and (you guessed it!) the submandibular glands.

JOT BOX

1.6 NEUROANATOMY AND NEUROSCIENCE

Brain regions

A succinct reminder of the five major regions of the brain.

Toddler's Messy Diapers Turn Yellow[8]

Toddler's	**T**elencephalon
Messy	**M**esencephalon
Diapers	**D**iencephalon
Turn	me**T**encephalon
Yellow	m**Y**encephalon

The cranial nerves

There are 12 cranial nerves, but how can you remember all their names, and with the right number? This helps but, again, use a German accent for best effect.[9]

On Old Olympus's Towering Top, A Finn Vith German Viewed A House

On	**O**lfactory	Ist cranial nerve
Old	**O**ptic	IInd cranial nerve
Olympus's	**O**culomotor	IIIrd cranial nerve
Towering	**T**rochlear	IVth cranial nerve
Top	**T**rigeminal	Vth cranial nerve
A	**A**bducens	VIth cranial nerve
Finn	**F**acial	VIIth cranial nerve
Vith	**V**estibulocochlear	VIIIth cranial nerve
German	**G**lossopharyngeal	IXth cranial nerve
Viewed	**V**agus	Xth cranial nerve
A	**A**ccessory	XIth cranial nerve
House	**H**ypoglossal	XIIth cranial nerve

8 Attributed to Debbie Rogers SGMS, 1990.
9 Modified from Browse N, Black J, Burnand KG, Thomas WEG (2005) *Browse's Introduction to Symptoms and Signs of Surgical Disease*, 4th edn. London: Arnold.

How can one remember which ones are *sensory* or which are *motor* or which are *both*? Here's an easy way and well-known device:

Some Say Marry Money But My Bride Says Big Balls Matter More

Some	**S**ensory	Ist cranial nerve
Say	**S**ensory	IInd cranial nerve
Marry	**M**otor	IIIrd cranial nerve
Money	**M**otor	IVth cranial nerve
But	**B**oth	Vth cranial nerve
My	**M**otor	VIth cranial nerve
Bride	**B**oth	VIIth cranial nerve
Says	**S**ensory	VIIIth cranial nerve
Big	**B**oth	IXth cranial nerve
Balls	**B**oth	Xth cranial nerve
Matter	**M**otor	XIth cranial nerve
More	**M**otor	XIIth cranial nerve

Alternatives

On Occasion Our Trusty Truck Acts Funny (Very Good Vehicle, Any How) – attributed to Arvinder Singh of Ipoh, Perak, Malaysia. But most students seem to prefer this anonymous (rude) version: Oh, Oh, Oh, To Touch and Feel Virgin Girls' Vaginas and Hymens.

Take a look at a really effective way to learn this list using the 'peg system' as described in Section III.

Dermatomes – made easier

Imagine (to switch on the right side of your brain) a four-legged mammal, rather than a biped – this makes understanding the dermatomes much easier. Now, start at C1 and work your way down.

- C1 to C4 go to the head, neck and shoulders.
- C5 to T1 'disappear' as they 'wander off' to innervate the upper limb.
- T4 supplies the nipples.
- T10 supplies the umbilicus (see below).
- T12 is the lowest abdominal dermatome.
- L1 to S1 go to the lower limb.
- S2 to S5 are the only ones left for the bottom end.

If you study the following diagram and transpose it to a person standing upright, you will see the way the dermatomes flow. Go with that flow!

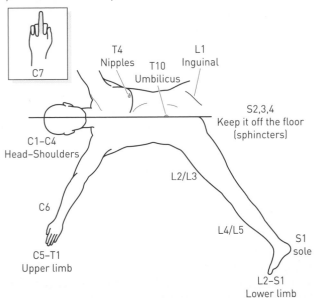

T4
Nipples
T10
Umbilicus
L1
Inguinal
C7
S2,3,4
Keep it off the floor
(sphincters)
C1–C4
Head–Shoulders
L2/L3
C6
L4/L5
S1
sole
C5–T1
Upper limb
L2–S1
Lower limb

NAUGHTY BIT

Remember T**4** = T **for** tits!

And more about the cervical dermatomes:

One cervical, two cervical, three cervical, four, down the upper limb to find any more
Hold out your arms like a crucifix, stick up your thumbs – you have C6
Now wiggle C7 – the middle finger to heaven
And easy to extrapolate – ring and little fingers are C8!

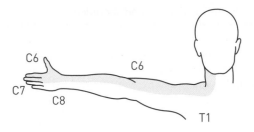

C6
C6
C7
C8
T1

T10 umbilicus

Did you know that the umbilicus is already *labelled* with its respective dermatome? Not convinced? Do I have to show you a diagram? OK here it is... *but for the rest of your life you will remember* that T10 innervates the umbilicus...

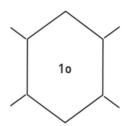

Some mnemonics for the dermatomes use the digit '1' instead of the letter 'I'. The dermatome to the axilla is T1 (remember the overlap of all the dermatomes). This is actually spelt out in the word 'armpit' like this:

T1 – armp**1T**

Dermatome L1 is spelt out in 'inguinal' as shown below. Thinking of this will also remind you that it is the **L**ast abdominal dermatome.

L1 – **1**nguina**L**

For L3, remember this is roughly where cowboys holster their guns, and remember this rhyme too:

L3 – goes to the medial knee

As for the first sacral nerve, S1, this supplies the little toes and the sole of the foot. Get it?!

S1 – **1 S**mall toe

or:

S1 – **S**o**1**e

Finally, S2 to S4 relate to the sphincters, thus:

S2, 3, 4 – keep it off the floor

You have now learned, with the minimum effort, most of the major dermatomes. Once you know a few of the key ones, you can extrapolate the rest. Remember that each dermatome overlaps with those above and below, which makes your revision even easier because you know the dermatome just above and below will be involved.

Another useful way of looking at the sacral dermatomes is summarized here:[10]

You stand on S1
Lie on S2
Sit on S3
Wipe S4
Poke S5 (rectum)

Review your knowledge of them with the song below, which ties all of this together. Remember that reviewing is a major key to success.

The dermatome song

One cervical, two cervical, three cervical, four, down the upper limb to find any more
Hold out your arms like a crucifix, stick up your thumbs – you have C6
Now wiggle C7 – the middle finger to heaven
And easy to extrapolate – ring and little fingers are C8!
T1 spelt in armp1T is – as for nipples, well T4 for tits
One dermatome ready labelled for us, T10 in the umbilicus!
L1 you know-it-all, 'cos it's spelt 1nguinaL
L3 to holster guns, you see, also goes to medial knee
L4 flows across the kneecap, but won't stop there, the busy chap,
It goes to make your bunion jingle – and with L5 the big toe tingle!
So to S1 and 1 small toe, a dermatome full of So1e
S2 on which you lie, S3 upon which you sit
S4 is what you wipe, S5 – put yer finger in it!

Perhaps not the most elegant of poems, but at least you know more dermatomes than you did 5 minutes ago!

Extraocular muscle innervation

Consider the following 'formula' to describe the innervation of these eye muscles.[11]

10 Contributed by Dr Laura Colvin.
11 Derived from Smith A (1972) *Irving's Anatomy Mnemonics*. Edinburgh: Churchill Livingstone.

LR6 (SO4) 3

LR6 **L**ateral **R**ecti   **6**th (VIth) cranial nerve (abducens)

SO4 **S**uperior **O**blique   **4**th (IVth) cranial nerve (trochlear)

3   All other extraocular   **3**rd (IIIrd) cranial nerve (oculomotor)

You now know the entire cranial innervation of the extraocular eye muscles – oh, you little genius! (And you can also remember that the *abducens* nerve *abducts* the eye.)

Facial (VII) nerve

Branches are:

Two Zebras Buggered My Cat

Two	**T**emporal
Zebras	**Z**ygomatic
Buggered	**B**uccal
My	**M**andibular
Cat	**C**ervical

NOTE: No cats (or zebras!) were harmed in the making of this book!

Alternative

The less risqué version is shown on the cover: Two Zebras Borrowed My Car.

SWOT BOX

The facial nerve exits the skull via the stylomastoid foramen then runs superficially within the parotid gland before dividing into five terminal branches which supply the muscles of facial expression. The mastoid process is not present at birth, thus a difficult labour or use of forceps may injure the facial nerve.

The superior part of the motor nucleus of the facial nerve has bilateral cortical innervation, hence the muscles of the upper part of the face have a bilateral nerve supply – which means that in an upper motor neuron lesion there is contralateral paralysis of the lower half of the face (though the patient will still be able to close their eyes and wrinkle their forehead muscles). With a lower motor neuron lesion (e.g. Bell's palsy) movement will be affected on the same side as the lesion. See also p. 104.

NAUGHTY BIT

What do the chorda tympanae (facial nerve branch) and the clitoris have in common?

(For the answer turn to the next page – any physical action will reinforce the information you are learning!)

Pain fibres

Here is a useful way to remember the differences between A and C pain fibres.

'**C**' fibres   Carry **C**rude touch
'**A**' fibres   Pain **A**rises **A**bruptly and is blocked by **A**sphyxia

SWOT BOX

C fibres are involved with pain that typically arises slowly and is poorly localized, often with a burning and unpleasant or disagreeable sensation.

A fibres are involved with pain that typically arises abruptly and is well localized, often with a sharp or prickling sensation. (Come to think of it, they have a lot in common with getting 'A' grades too.)

Ventral and dorsal spinal columns

It is easy to remember that the grey ventral columns are motor.

Motor   The **motor** is in the **front** (ventral) of most cars!
Sensory   **S**ensory modalities are dor**s**al

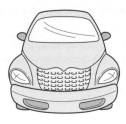

ANSWER: They both supply taste to the anterior two-thirds of the tongue. (Awful, isn't it! And anonymous – not surprisingly!)

Also, to remind you of the sensory modalities (joint position, vibration, pressure, touch) which are in the dorsal (posterior) spinal column – take a look at Julie's Visible Panty Line.

Julie's Visible Panty Line

Julie's	Joint position
Visible	Vibration
Panty	Pressure
Line	Light touch

Vestibulocochlear (VIII) nerve – a test

A test for the vestibular division of the VIIIth nerve involves pouring cold or warm water into the external auditory meatus (ear hole) to bring about a temperature change. This temperature change affects the movement of endolymph in the semicircular ducts, and stimulates the hair cells (movement sensors) of the cristae. This in turn stimulates the vestibular nerve via the oculogyric nuclei in the brainstem, and causes nystagmus. Cold water causes nystagmus in the direction of the opposite eye; warm water causes it in the direction of the same eye. You can remember this with the COWS mnemonic.

COWS

C–O	Cold water – Opposite eye
W–S	Warm water – Same eye

SWOT BOX

Remember, the conventional direction of nystagmus is considered to be the direction of the 'quick' flick. In nystagmus, the eye wanders off, out of control. Your neurology attempts to correct it by flicking the eye back into position, so it can fixate on the object being looked at.

Wear a smile and have friends
Wear a frown and have wrinkles

George Eliot

BIOCHEMISTRY

These tips and suggestions will help with your biochemistry revision. Try this first:

PRE-QUIZ

1 How many rings are there in the adenine nucleotide?
2 Which are the pyrimidine nucleotide bases?
3 How many hydrogen bonds are there between guanine and cytosine?
4 What are the four fates of pyruvate?
5 Can you draw the Lineweaver–Burke plot of competitive inhibition?
6 How many essential amino acids are there? Can you name them?

Amino acids – essential

There are 20 amino acids in all but only 10 are *essential*. Eight of them are essential *always*, and two of them (histidine and arginine) are essential *only* in specific cases. The names of all 10 can be remembered by the following phrase.

I Saw, He Phoned at 3:09 and Met Licentious Argentines – Lucy, Tracey and Val

I saw	**Iso**leucine
He	**H**istidine
Phoned at	**Ph**enylalanine
3:09	**Thre**onine
Met	**Met**hionine
Licentious	**Lys**ine
Argentines	**Arg**inine
Lucy	**Leuc**ine
Tracey and	**Tr**yptophan
Val	**Val**ine

Amino acids – structure

The amino acids with *positive side chains* are given by HAL.

HAL

H	**H**istidine
A	**A**rginine
L	**L**ysine

Although the *R* group varies, you will probably know that *all* amino acids have this structure in common:

$$H_3N - \overset{\overset{\displaystyle R}{|}}{\underset{|}{C}} - COOH$$

Here are some handy aides for recalling the details about the structures of individual amino acids.

Glycine **R = H (H**ydrogen)

The simplest amino acid. We don't bother to write the letter **H** on chemical structures because the marked ends indicate hydrogen. So glycine's structure is the same as the above with the **R** bit left blank

Alanine **R = CH$_3$ (Me**thyl group)

Hence 'It's all about **Me**, me, me... it's all-a-mine!' (*all-a-mine* rhymes with alanine)

Valine **R = V-shaped group**

The V-shape is shown in the diagram below. This makes it so easy – just stick a **V** up your **R**!

$$H_2N \diagup \overset{\overset{\displaystyle R}{|}}{\underset{|}{C}} - COOH \quad = \quad H_2N \diagup \overset{\overset{\displaystyle V}{|}}{\underset{|}{C}} - COOH$$
Valine

Cystine **R = contains C-S (S**ulfur attached to Carbon)

The clue is in the name Cy**S**tine

Leucine	**R = looks like λ**
	The Greek letter *lambda* (see below) gives us an 'L' sound for leucine

$$\text{Leucine: -}\quad R = \quad \begin{array}{c} | \\ -C- \\ | \\ C \\ \diagup\diagdown \\ -C-\ -C- \\ |\quad | \end{array} \quad \text{or } λ$$

Methionine	**R = C–C–S–C**
	What sounds will remind you of that? How about *cake-suck* or *Coxsackie's* (a virus)? How about a phrase like *methionine makes coke suck* (–C–C–S–C)
Arginine	**R = Pr–N–CNN** (**P**ropyl, **C**arbon, **N**itrogen)
	Say *Argentina prayin' for CNN* to remind you of this side group
Serine	**R = CH2OH** (methanol)
	Think of a *searin'* pain caused by drinking methanol
Threonine	**R = EtOH** (ethanol)
	Threonine has three oxygen atoms (*three-O*) and nine H atoms (*-nine*) – convenient, eh!
Proline	**R = ring-shaped** **N**itrogen-containing ring
	R is shaped like a **P**entago**N** with **N**itrogen in one corner – draw it out for yourself

Base-pairing

You will remember that the **nucleic acid** purine *only* pairs with a pyrimidine, giving a constant three-ring diameter to DNA. Use this rule:

AT the GEC

AT the	**A**denine only pairs with **T**hymine
GEC	**G**uanine links (via three hydrogen bonds) with **C**ytosine

This is ridiculously easy to remember if you think of the General Electric Company, the GEC, and if you know the E represents three hydrogen bonds:

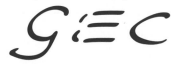

The cell cycle

The five phases of cell mitosis are encompassed by the IPMAT mnemonic.

IPMAT

I	**I**nterphase
P	**P**rophase
M	**M**etaphase
A	**A**naphase
T	**T**elophase

The many stages of meiosis are remembered using PMAT–PMAT.

PMAT-PMAT

P	**P**rophase 1
M	**M**etaphase 1
A	**A**naphase 1
T	**T**elophase 1
P_2	**P**rophase 2
M_2	**M**etaphase 2
A_2	**A**naphase 2
T_2	**T**elophase 2

Enzyme inhibition

The Lineweaver–Burk plot is a graph showing competitive inhibition between two enzymes (graph, below right). You can remember this by visualizing two crossed swords – in competition. In non-competitive inhibition, they do not cross.

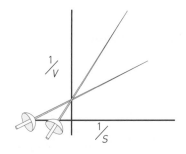

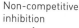

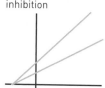

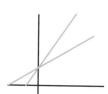

Huckle's rule of spatial stability

As you know, spatial stability is associated with six electrons. Well, it just so happens there are precisely the same number of letters in the word Huckle.

6 electrons **6** letters in Huckle

Lipids

Very-low-density lipoproteins (VLDLs) carry endogenous triglycerides from the liver to cells for storage for metabolism – these are the bad ones! High-density lipoproteins (HDLs) carry cholesterol away from the peripheral cells to liver for excretion – these are the good ones! Remember the difference like this:

HDL	**H** for **H**eroes
VLDL	**V** for **V**illains

Ortho, para and meta substitutions

Ortho means on position 2 of the aromatic ring. *Meta* means on position 3. *Para* is at position 4 and parallel to the carbon at position 1. To remember this easily, remember:

Or-two met-a-tree para-four

Or-two	**Ortho-2**
Meta a tree	**Met-3**
Para-four	**Para-4** parallel to C1

Purine and pyrimidine nucleic acids

Nucleic acids are made up of a base, a five-carbon sugar and a phosphate group. The bases are either purines (two-ringed) adenine and guanine, or pyrimidines. The latter are the single-ringed thymine and cytosine (or uracil in RNA). Within the nucleic acid chain, a pyrimidine always links with a purine and vice versa. So a DNA double-helix is *always* three rings wide.

All Girls Are Pure and Wear Bras

All	**A**denine
Girls are	**G**uanine
Pure	**P**urines

And to help you remember their structures:

Purines are two-ringed structures...
... and so are bras!

This leaves the single-ringed Pyrimidines, Thymine and Cytosine. You can try to visualize Pies, Tyres or Cytes (cells) to remind you of single-ring shapes, or perhaps a 'seat' for cytosine. Get the picture?

Penser, c'est voir
(To think is to see)

Louis Lambert

Pyruvate metabolism

The four fates of pyruvate are given by GALA and are shown in the diagram below.

GALA

G	**G**lucose
A	**A**lanine
L	**L**actate
A	**A**cetyl coenzyme A

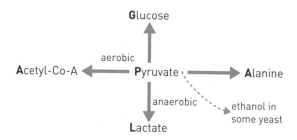

Redox reactions

This is an old school favourite – another anonymous one – about the loss of electrons in redox reactions.

OIL RIG

O	**O**xidation
I	**I**s
L	**L**oss
R	**R**eduction
I	**I**s
G	**G**ain

Stereoisomers

Cis molecules have both their R groups on the same side of a double bond, but *trans* molecules have them on opposite sides. Remember:

Both on 'cis' side

The urea cycle

Several students claim that this anonymous mnemonic actually helped them learn the urea cycle. There is no accounting for taste!

Ordinarily Careless Crappers Are Also Frivolous About Urination

Ordinarily	**O**rnithine
Careless	**C**arbamoyl
Crappers	**C**itrulline
Are	**A**spartate
Also	**A**rginosuccinate

Frivolous   **F**umarate

About   **A**rginine

Urination   **U**rea

However, the biochemical cycles be learnt by use of loci or peg mnemonics. See more on advanced mnemonics in Section III.

Vitamins – Bs

There are eight B vitamins. Remember:

B looks like number **8**

Namely:

B1, B2, B3, B5, B6, B7, B9, B12

Most are enzyme co-factors or are involved with metabolism. The B vitamins are water-soluble. The fat-soluble vitamins are given below.

Vitamins – fat-soluble

ADEK

A	Vitamin **A**
D	Vitamin **D**
E	Vitamin **E**
K	Vitamin **K**

JOT BOX

PHYSIOLOGY

The first qualification for a physician is hopefulness
James Little (1836–1885)

How good is your knowledge of physiology right now?

Anterior pituitary hormones

The **six anterior pituitary hormones** are thyroid-stimulating hormone (TSH), growth hormone (GH), the two gonadotrophins (follicle-stimulating hormone (FSH) and luteinizing hormone (LH)), prolactin (PRL) and adrenocorticotrophic hormone (ACTH).

Those Giant Gonads Prolong the Action

THo**S**e	**TSH**
Giant	**G**H
Gonads	FSH/LH
PRo**L**ong the	**PRL**
ACTion	**ACT**H

Blood pressure

'BP Copper' is a neat reminder of the relationship between **arterial blood pressure** (BP), cardiac output (CO) and peripheral resistance (PR).

BP Copper
$$BP = CO \times PR$$

If you ever get confused about whether **systolic pressure** or **diastolic pressure** is higher, think of 'S' for *squeezing* which is what the heart does during systole – hence giving a *higher* reading.

Systolic pressure = **S**queezing
Diastolic = **D**ilating heart or **D** for down

Canal of Schlemm

The canal is a space at the sclerocorneal junction. It drains the aqueous fluid away from the anterior chamber. Any increased resistance to this flow will cause a rise in intraocular pressure (IOP). Here's a handy description:

C.C.C.P.
C	**C**onstriction of the
C	**C**ircular muscle opens up the
C	**C**anal of Schlemm
P	**P**arasympathetically

SWOT BOX

Friedrich S. Schlemm (1795–1858) was Professor of Anatomy in Berlin. He was **over 21** years old when he discovered the canal. By a freak coincidence, an IOP of **over 21** mmHg is a sign of glaucoma. Gotcha...! Now for the rest of your medical career you will know that an intraocular pressure **over 21** is a sign of glaucoma – whether or not you wanted to!

JOT BOX

Ejaculation

Is ejaculation mediated by parasympathetic or sympathetic nerves? If you think of the erection as pointing and the ejaculation as shooting, this makes perfect sense.[1] (Surely you don't need a diagram for this one.)

Point and Shoot

Point   **P**arasympathetic
Shoot   **S**ympathetic

Excretory organs

Recalling the five main excretory organs is a SKILL well worth knowing!

SKILL

S   **S**kin
K   **K**idneys
I   **I**ntestines
L   **L**iver
L   **L**ungs

Fluid compartments

This one needs a little bit of thought (stay calm – it's not too much). You need to say to yourself '1-2-3-30-45 if pit'. It works something like this:

1-2-3-30-45 .... If Pit

12 litres   **IF**   **I**nterstitial **F**luid
3 litres (plasma)   **P**   **P**lasma
30 litres (inside cells)   **I**   **I**nside cells
45 litres (total body water)   **T**   **T**otal body water

Do have a go. Contributed by an anonymous medical student, several others have found it helpful. Write it out a few times *now* and you will remember it. Writing will reinforce a motor memory and sensory pathway to strengthen the visual stimulus of the above.

---

1 With acknowledgement to P. McCoubrie and M. Jones, St George's Hospital Medical School, London, 1990.

Heart sounds

The first heart sound (S1) is made up of a mitral component (M1) and a tricuspid (T1) component (in order of valve closure). The second (S2) is made up of A2 (aortic) followed by the pulmonary valve closure (P2). This gives a sequence from S1 to S2 of M1–T1–A2–P2.

You will find this sequence easy to learn with 'Mighty Ape'.

Mighty Ape

Migh**T**y   **M**1 **T**1
APe   **A**2 **P**2

See page 83 for more on heart sounds and murmurs.

Immunoglobulins

There are five classes of immunoglobulins – IgG, IgA, IgM, IgE and IgD.

GAMED

immunoglobulin **G**
immunoglobulin **A**
immunoglobulin **M**
immunoglobulin **E**
immunoglobulin **D**

Each has four polypeptide chains – two heavy and two light. These chains are held together by disulfide (**S–S**) bonds. Heavy chains are specific to each class of Ig. IgM is produced first in the immune response. IgG appears later as the IgM level falls. This secondary response of IgG is due to activation of long-lived B lymphocytes on repeated exposure to the antigen. The secondary response is quicker and greater. Remember:

Ig**M**   **IM**mediately produced
Ig**G**   **G**reater response

JOT BOX

Khalid's guide to the sarcomere

1. Draw two 'Z lines' – the borders of our 'Zarcomere'.

2. Draw an 'M' line in the Middle.

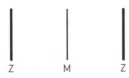

3. Add a dArk 'A' bAnd.

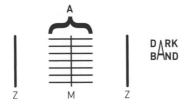

D∧RK
B∧ND

4. What's left must be the light 'I' zone.

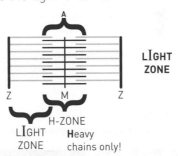

LIGHT
ZONE

H-ZONE
LIGHT   Heavy
ZONE   chains only!

Simple!

PHARMACOLOGY

This chapter will be useful in both your physiology and pharmacology. The section on receptors is relevant to your understanding of drug modes of action.

PRE-QUIZ

1. Are beta-1 receptors found predominantly in the lung or in the heart?
2. Can you name two non-adrenergic non-cholinergic neurotransmitters?
3. Which muscarinic receptors are more common in the brain?
4. What are the effects of beta blockers on the lungs?
5. Is the above mediated by the sympathetic or parasympathetic system?
6. Is phenytoin used in the treatment of petit mal epilepsy?
7. Which prostaglandins dilate blood vessels?
8. What is the quadruple therapy of tuberculosis?

4.1 RECEPTOR REVISION

Adrenoreceptors

In general, **alpha-stimulation** causes constriction of smooth muscles. A handy way to remember this is to imagine that the Greek letter α is made of rope, so when the two ends are pulled it forms a tight knot.

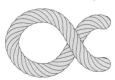

In general, beta-stimulation 'makes 'em bigger', meaning they cause the dilation of smooth muscles in structures such as the bronchioles, uterus, blood vessels. A good memory jogger is therefore:

> **B**eta makes 'em **B**igger

And what about beta receptors in the **heart and lungs**? It's easy to learn which subtype predominates in each. The heart has predominantly beta-1 receptors, and the lungs have mainly beta-2, and of course you have one heart and two lungs. So:

One Heart Two Lungs

One heart	Beta **one**
Two lungs	Beta **two**

Could it be any easier?

Catecholamines

The three stages of **noradrenaline (norepinephrine) synthesis** are: tyrosine → DOPA (dihydroxy-L-phenylalanine) → dopamine → norepinephrine. Although it's a bit outdated now, here's a handy reminder:

Tired Dopes Do Nada

Tired	**T**yrosine
DOPes	**DOP**A
Do	**D**opamine
Nada	**Norad**re**na**line

Alternative

Tiresome Dopes Dominate Norway.

The **enzymes** involved in these three steps are hydroxylase, decarboxylase, and beta-hydroxylase. If the hydroxyl component is represented by the chemical formula (OH), you can use this to remind you:

Hide De Ho

Hi**De**	**Hyd**roxylase
De	**De**carboxylase
HO	Beta-**OH**-lase (hydroxylase)

Catecholamine metabolism is via a *cytoplasmic* enzyme called catechol-O-methyltransferase (or COMT) and two *mitochondrial* enzymes called monoamine oxidase A and monoamine oxidase B – the MAOs. Think:

Cytoplasm   **C**OMT
Mitochondria   **M**AO

Muscarinic receptors and blockers

There are five subtypes of **muscarinic receptor** (M_1 to M_5). They are usually neuroeffectors for the parasympathetic system, peripherally, where they are found in smooth muscle and glands.

MSG

M	**M**uscarinic (receptors peripherally are in...)
S	**S**mooth muscles (and...)
G	**G**lands

They are also very important centrally – especially the M_1 subtype. Generally they work by reducing cAMP (cyclic adenosine triphosphate). M_1 receptors are the most important and most widely expressed muscarinic receptors in the brain. M_2 receptors slow the heart down. M_3 receptors are the most important for bladder contraction.

This all ties together in the 'Muscarinic receptor song'.

Muscarinic receptor song

Muscle-bound men are a **little camp**	**Decreases cAMP**
My **big secret** makes you damp	**Increases secretions/** contraction
'Coz...	
M3 makes me **pee**!	**Bladder** contraction
M2 **slows the heart**, dude	**Bradycardia**
M1 motorway – the **northern route**!	North is 'up' – like the **brain**!

Applied mnemonics – the actions of atropine

Once you know the actions of the parasympathetic system you can work out most of the actions of atropine, which is a **muscarinic blocker**.

Starting with the CNS with all those M_1 (northern route) receptors, atropine is excitatory. Not surprisingly, atropine was used to make women appear more beautiful (bella donnas) when they took the stuff (from the deadly nightshade plant *Atropa belladonna*) because it dilated their pupils – muscarinic receptors constrict the pupils. Remember C.C.C.P. – Constriction of Circular muscle opens up the Canal of Schlemm Parasympathetically. So, if you block it, the pupils widen.

Moving on to the **heart,** we know M_2 slows the heart so, if atropine blocks this action (of the vagus nerve), the heart will... speed up, leaving the beta-1 receptors working just fine and without any opposite slowing-down effect of the parasympathetics.

This brings us to the **lungs**. If the parasympathetic system constricts things, then blocking it should help here – and so we have **ipratropium**, derived from atropine (as the name suggests) as a cholinergic muscarinic receptor blocker – used as an inhaler in asthma and chronic airflow limitation to assist breathing.

Now to the **GI** side of things. If M receptors predominantly increase gastric and bladder motility, then if we block this effect with atropine maybe it will slow down diarrhoea? Enter co-phenotrope, said to be especially formulated to reduce gut motility for the troops in Vietnam (trade name Lomotil), which contains our buddy atropine.

Stimulating M_3 makes you pee – so atropine should have the opposite effect and reduce bladder contractions. Thus, anticholinergics are used to stabilize the bladder and treat incontinence.

HOT HINT: Using the same process as above, and working head downwards, extrapolate the actions of drugs on the various organ systems.

NANC transmitters

The NANC (non-adrenergic non-cholinergic) neurotransmitters include nitrous oxide (NO) and the catecholamine dopamine.

Nancy Boys Are No Dopes
NANCy boys are   **N**on-**A**drenergic **N**on-**C**holinergics
NO   **N**itrous **O**xide
DOPes   **D**opamine

Parasympathetic system

Here is a useful summary of the **gastrointestinal functions** of the parasympathetic nervous system:

Periods Must Increase Secret Stomach Cramps

Periods	**P**arasympathetic system neuroeffector junctions are all...
Must	**M**uscarinic and...
Increase	**I**ncrease...
Secret	**S**ecretions of the...
Stomach	**G**astrointestinal system and...
Cramps	**G**astric motility

Other systemic parasympathetic system effects are covered by this neat phrase:

Decreased Arti's by Bringing Brad Pitt

Decreased	Reduction or constriction of...
Arti's by	**Art**erioles
Bringing	**Br**onchioles
Brad	**(Brad**y)cardia
Pitt	**P**upils

Alternative

Bringing Brad's Pills Decreased Arti's.

RAPID REVISION

Erection is mediated **P**arasympathetically (**P**ointing) and ejaculation is mediated **S**ympathetically (**S**hooting) system (see p. 41).

From the central nervous system the first stop for all nerves are always nicotinic receptors. After that, all **parasympathetic neuroeffector junctions** are *muscarinic* – thus the final stop is always muscarinic. Thus their path is spinal cord → nicotinic → muscarinic.

Pat likes S 'n' M

Pat likes	**P**arasympathetic (nerves from the...)
S	**S**pinal cord (go via...)
N	**N**icotinic (then...)
M	**M**uscarinic

Zero-order kinetics

It is useful to know some drugs with zero-order kinetics.

Constantly Aspiring To Phone Ethan

Constantly	(zero-order kinetics)
Aspiring	**Asp**irin
To **PH**one	**Ph**enytoin
ETHan	**Eth**anol

JOT BOX

4.2 PHARMACOLOGY AND THERAPEUTICS

Adrenaline (Epipen)

'Pattern of 3s'

Dose for acute anaphylaxis is **300 micrograms** for children > **30** kg. Can be repeated after 5–15 minutes as necessary.

6-Aminopenicillamic acid – structure

6-APA – the basis of the penicillins!

1. Draw a house:

2. Add a garage and smoke from the chimney:

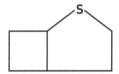

3. Add an outdoor aerial and a garden fence:

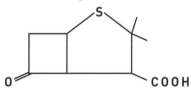

4. Stick on an amide group:

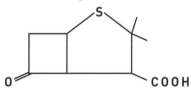

Congratulations!

Antiepileptics

Current treatment of **petit mal epilepsy** involves use of **valproate** and **ethosuximide**. According to the observation of the 'paradoxical Ps', if a drug name starts with a **P**, then it ain't used for **P**etit mal epilepsy!

Paradoxical Ps

NOT for **P**etit mal:

Phenytoin

Primidone

Phenobarbital

SWOT BOX

Petit mal, or absence seizures, are brief, generalized seizures. They have a particular spike-wave pattern of about 3 Hz on EEG. They usually occur in children aged 4–12 and are characterized by lapses of concentration and rhythmic movements of eyelids and hands. There is rapid return to full consciousness without retrograde amnesia or confusion. Many patients later develop generalized tonic–clonic seizures.

The names of **antiepileptic drugs** are interesting. **Phenytoin** is one of the barbiturates, named after a waitress in Munich called *Barbara* as well as *urea* (according to Sharpless,[1] Barbara even supplied some of the raw materials required). The antiepileptic **vigabatrin** was named after its mode of action, which is inhibition of gamma-aminobutyric acid (GABA)-transferase. The anticonvulsant drug **clobazam** has a name that sounds like the action of knocking patients out (say it quickly!). The analgesic **dolobid** derives from *dolor* (pain of inflammation) and the abbreviation for a twice daily dose *bid*. **Lasix** is furosemide, and it was named thus because it 'lasts six hours'.

JOT BOX

1 Sharpless SK (1965) The barbiturates. In: *The Pharmacological Basis of Therapeutics*, 3rd edn. New York: Macmillan, pp. 105–28.

Antituberculosis drugs

This consists of triple or quadruple therapy – RIP or RIP(E).

RIP(E)

R	**R**ifampicin
I	**I**soniazid
P	**P**yrazinamide
(E)	**(E**thambutol**)**

Poor compliance to this therapy is best reduced by using combination tablets (such as rifampicin + isoniazid), urine testing for rifampicin (*Prescriber's Journal* 2000: 40(1)) as well as by DOT:

DOT

D	**D**irectly
O	**O**bserved
T	**T**reatment

SWOT BOX

The **usual regimen** consists of minimum 2 months of RIPE followed by another 4 months of rifampicin + isoniazid (in adults, children, pregnant and breastfeeding women). Depending on the results of cultures, it may be necessary to increase either one or both phases of treatment.

With **CNS involvement** the full course is usually longer (2 months RIPE + 8 months rifampicin + isoniazid).

HIV patients are usually given the standard regimen, unless there is multidrug-resistant disease. Liver p450 enzyme induction by rifampicin may make protease inhibitors ineffective, so an alternative retroviral or anti-TB regimen may have to be used.

The **peripheral neuropathy of isoniazid** may be prevented in those at risk (e.g. in HIV, diabetics, chronic renal failure, malnutrition) with 10 mg daily of vitamin B6.

Atorvastatin

Statins are generally given only at night because cholesterol synthesis is at its highest overnight. Atorvastatin is the only statin that can be taken at any time because of its long duration of action. Remember it like this:

At or any time

| At Or | **Ator**vastatin |
| any time | **day or night** |

Beta blockers

This is your first session with spatial mnemonics, covered in much more detail in Section III. We shall use them to learn about beta blockers.

Spatial mnemonics are a little more advanced than simple mnemonics. Such 'spatial' or 'loci' learning systems involve linking something you need to learn fast to something you already know now – in this case your own body!

Use exaggerated link-association as described in Section III. The very act of reading the whole story that follows will help you.

A good system is to start at the head (the CNS) and work downwards. We will use propanolol as our 'typical' beta blocker. Remember to make your mental images bold, multisensory and exaggerated.

Now, if you are up for it, let's roll...

Effects of propanolol

| CENTRAL NERVOUS SYSTEM | **Propanolol** causes fatigue and depression | *Imagine you are feeling really wonderful and energetic and a '**pro**' tries to block this by 'interacting' with your head (brain)* |
| EYES | Dilates pupils by blocking the sympathetic system so the parasympathetic takes over (e.g. **tim**olol eye drops treat open-angle glaucoma) | *If you know somebody called **Tim**, imagine him putting drops in your eyes* |

HEART	Blocks beta-1 receptors so the heart slows down as the parasympathetic system takes over (remember, *the vagus nerve (M2) slows the heart, dude*)	*You might think of a heart-stopping heartthrob called Brad, for example*
PERIPHERAL VASCULAR SYSTEM	Vasoconstriction. Remember beta makes 'em bigger. Well, if you block this, then the opposite happens, resulting in **freezing** cold extremities	*'Brrrr... Brr... Brad!'*
LUNGS	**Broncho**constriction beta-2 effect (remember, *2 lungs*)	*Imagine something like a wheezing bucking bronco on your chest*
MUSCULOSKELETAL	Reduces tremor	*That pro is calming things down*
METABOLIC	Raises cholesterol	*Hey, you do some work here!*
KINETICS	It is protein bound with a short half-life of 4 hours	

Once you have a spatial sequence to your liking, pencil it down and work through it a few times in your head. You will find that you will remember much more material this way, and it is significantly quicker to review the night before your exam. You can use any well-known objects, structures and people with this technique, like your own house for alpha blockers, your porch for penicillin, and your kitchen for the Krebs cycle!

Curare

Curare is a competitive inhibitor which blocks nicotinic receptors. Simply put:

Curare = **C**ompetitive inhibitor

Loop diuretics

Furosemide and **bumetanide** are both loop diuretics. The **loop** of Henle is **U-shaped** like the letter they both share (U) so this is a helpful reminder.

U-shape (loop of Henle)

fUrosemide
bUmetanide

Prostaglandins

Prostaglandin-1 and **prostaglandin-2** are vasodilators, with their main effects on *arteries*. **Prostaglandin-A** and **prostaglandin-E** are vasodilators, with their main effects on *veins*.

Again substituting the digit '1' with the letter 'I' means you can think of:

DIlAtE

DI	**1**/2
LATE	**A/E**

Sympathomimetic amines

Directly acting sympathomimetic amines can be recalled using the mnemonic: I Saw Ape Naked.

I Saw Ape Naked

I Saw	**IS**oprenaline
A**PE**	**EP**inephrine
Naked	**N**or**A**drenaline (or **N**or**E**pinephrine)

Alternatives

Try this one: I Saw Adrian Naked (where Adrian stands for adrenaline). Or: Directly I-saw Ape Naked and Acted Sympathetically.

MICROBIOLOGY AND INFECTIOUS DISEASES

When you have read this chapter, you will be able to tackle the following with ease:

PRE-QUIZ

1 What are the complications of mumps?
2 Is *Neisseria* a Gram-negative or Gram-positive organism?
3 Does *Shigella* have flagella for motility?
4 Can you name some non-lactose fermenters?
5 What are the features of syphilis?

Cytomegalovirus

The abbreviation for cytomegalovirus is CMV, which – somewhat conveniently – is an acronym for the main symptoms of the disease.

CMV

C	**C**olitis
M	**M**outh dysphagia and oesophogeal ulceration
V	**V**isual problems (retinitis)

Diarrhoea in kids

Endemic **viral diarrhoea** in children is predominantly associated with rotaviruses, adenoviruses, caliciviruses and astroviruses. These are represented by:

Aiden strokes Cali's rottweiler

Aiden	**Aden**oviruses
Strokes	a**Stro**viruses
Cali's	**Cali**civiruses
Rottweiler	**Rot**aviruses

Mumps

Moping about mumps is a sure-fire way of remembering its four main symptoms.

MOPE

M	**M**eningism
O	**O**rchitis/**O**ophoritis
P	**P**arotitis/**P**ancreatitis/**P**aramyxovirus
E	**E**ncephalitis

SWOT BOX

Mumps is an air-borne **paramyxovirus**. It is also spread by direct contact with body fluids. Uncommon in adults, it is often subclinical in children. Usually salivary gland inflammation is the principal manifestation (e.g. uni- or bilateral parotitis).

Complications include epididymo-orchitis, oophoritis, meningo-encephalitis and pancreatitis. Mumps meningitis is usually benign, with vomiting, neck rigidity, lethargy, headache, photophobia, convulsions, and abdominal pain and fever.

Neisseria – negative sugar

Microbiologists use cultures containing glucose and maltose to differentiate between the negative cocci *Neisseria meningitides* and *Neisseria gonorrhoea*. This is called the sugar fermentation test. *Neisseria gonorrhoea* ferments glucose only, while *Neisseria meningitides* ferments glucose and maltose.

*N. **g**onorrhoea*	Ferments **g**lucose only
*N. **m**eningitides*	Ferments **m**altose as well

RNA viruses

It might only be a coincidence, but most RNA viruses start with the letter 'R' – like **r**habdovirus, **r**eovirus, **r**otavirus, and **r**hinovirus. Yet another coincidence is that drugs containing the letters '**vir**' are often anti**vir**al – like Retro**vir**, Zo**vir**ax and Vecta**vir**. So in general:

RNA viruses   Start with the letter **R**
Anti**VIR**al drugs   Contain the letters **VIR**

Salmonella and *Shigella*

Both these organisms are important in food poisoning. They are both non-lactose fermenters. *Salmonella* are flagellate organisms and are motile; in contrast, *Shigella* have no flagella and are therefore non-motile. But can you remember which is the motile one when you are under pressure? Well, you can easily – if you think of a salmon and remember that it is motile – so is *Salmonella*!

*Salmon*ella are motile like **salmon**

Try drawing a picture of a salmon(ella).

You can learn all the **non-lactose fermenters** with **SSPP**.

SSPP

S	*S*almonella
S	*S*higella
P	**P**seudomonas
P	**P**roteus

Syphilis

Syphilis is a subacute to chronic infectious disease caused by the spirochete *Treponema pallidum*. Doctors used to treat it with *quacksalver*, a cream containing mercury. The word *quack* derives from this. Quacksalver became *quicksilver*, which is still a synonym for the element mercury. A popular joke when this disease hit Europe was 'You spend one night with Venus – and six months with Mercury'!

A small red papule or crusted erosion called a **chancre** appears at the site of inoculation as a painless primary lesion, which often breaks down with a serous exudate. The tertiary stage occurs after many years, as neurosyphilis, with neurological symptoms that include **tabes dorsalis** and **delusions of grandeur**. Tabes in neurosyphilis is a progressive degeneration of the posterior columns, posterior roots and ganglia of the spinal cord, giving symptoms such as lightning pains, ataxia, urinary incontinence, optic atrophy, Charcot's joints, hypotonia and hyper-reflexia. Transmission may also be *in utero* (see TORCH'S infections on p. 124), leading to various congenital manifestations, including anterior bowing of the mid-portion of the tibia (**sabre shin**). This is a late congenital sign, seen less frequently now due to treatment with penicillin.

Here is a great summary of what the condition involves:[1]

> There was a young lad from Bombay
> Whose **chancre** just wouldn't fade away
> Well, apart from his **tabes**
> and **sabre**-legged babies
> Now he **thinks** he's Fay Wray!

SWOT BOX

Syphilis was the name of a shepherd infected with the disease in a poem of Fracastorius (1530), perhaps derived from the Greek *syn* (together) and *philein* (to love). It appeared in Europe at the siege of Naples (1495). As it spread through the continent, the French called it the Italian disease, the Italians called it the Spanish disease, and the Spanish called it the English disease...[2,3]

NAUGHTY BIT

Why is an Argyll Robertson pupil like a prostitute?

Because it accommodates but doesn't react!

JOT BOX

1 Contributed by Dr Bobby Bhartia, SGUL.
2 From Gertz SD, Gaithersburg MD (1996) *Liebman's Neuroanatomy Made Easy and Understandable*, 3rd edn. Aspen Publishers, and *Dorling's Medical Dictionary*, 28th edn. Philadelphia: WB Saunders.
3 Kirstin Harper (Emory University, Atlanta, USA, 2008) has described how syphilis may have originated in South America (Columbus returned from the New World in 1492).

Tuberculosis

RAPID REVISION

Therapy of TB was discussed on p. 52. Initial treatment is with triple or quadruple therapy – with RIP or RIP(E) – with Rifampicin, Isoniazid, Pyrazinamide (and Ethambutol). Further treatment is with just rifampicin and isoniazid. Patient compliance can be problem.

JOT BOX

SECTION

II

CLINICAL SPECIALTIES

CHEMICAL PATHOLOGY

The physician… has to know the cause of the ailment before he can cure it
Mocius (c.470–390 BC)

By the time you've mused through this section, you will be able to tackle these:

PRE-QUIZ

1 How many causes of low plasma sodium can you think of?
2 Can you think of any causes of raised potassium?
3 Can you list three causes of lowered serum phosphate?
4 What does a low plasma T4 level with a low level of thyroid-stimulating hormone suggest?
5 What about a low plasma T4 and a high thyroid-stimulating hormone level?
6 What are the features of Conn's syndrome?

Addison's disease

Addison's is the syndrome of adrenal insufficiency. To remind yourself of this,

ADDison's due to **AD**renal **D**eficiency

(**NOTE: C**ushing's (see p. 92) is caused by too much **C**ortisol.)

Alkaline phosphatase – raised

Big (= *raised*) Plate of Liver and Kidney Beans

Plate of	**P**lacental alkaline phosphatase in pregnancy
Liver and	**L**iver disease (?cholestasis)
Kidney	**K**idney (renal) failure
Beans	**B**one disease (isoenzyme)

The isoenzyme is related to osteoblast activity, especially in Paget's disease, child growth, healing, metastases, osteomalacia and hyperparathyroidism.

'Hi alk, phos alone... think bone!'

SWOT BOX

Alkaline phosphatase (AP) levels are elevated in various conditions, most commonly with hepatobiliary or bone pathology.

If only AP is raised (with all other liver enzymes and/or GGT being normal), then high AP is most likely due to bone pathology, e.g. osteomalacia, vitamin D deficiency, bony mets, fractures, renal osteodystrophy.

Bilirubin – unconjugated

Remember the causes with this simple memory jogger.

Uncle Gilbert's Creaky Home

Uncle	**Unc**onjugated due to...
Gilbert's	**Gilbert's**
Creaky	**Cr**igler–Najjar
Home	**H**aemolysis

Conn's syndrome

The important features of Conn's are **low renin**, **high aldosterone**, **alkalosis**, **low potassium** and **hypertension**, and common presentations are high **blood pressure**, **fatigue**, **muscle pain** and **headaches**. The syndrome is named after J.W. Conn, a US physician. Here is a good ditty for getting these main features into your memory.

An **alkalotic** young **CON**man named Mervin   **Alkalosis**, **Con**n's syndrome

Had **headache** 'cos there was **no rainin'**   **Headaches** **No rennin**

With no **pot** to grow   Low **pot**assium

High **pressure**, you know   High blood **pressure**

High aldosterone was making him **paining**!   **High aldosterone** and **muscle cramps**

Hyponatraemia

For the causes of low plasma sodium, use this memorable phrase.

Adding Sid's Hair Dye Creates Seriously Low Volume

Adding	**Add**ison's
Sid's	**SI**ADH (syndrome of inappropriate ADH)
Hair	**H**ypothyroid
Dye	**D**iuretics (especially thiazides)
Creates	**C**arbamazepine
Seriously	**S**SRIs (selective serotonin reuptake inhibitors)
Low **volume**	**Volume** depreciation (postural drop in blood pressure)

Plasma phosphate – raised

Causes of raised plasma phosphate are renal failure, delayed separation of sample and vitamin D excess. Here is a mnemonic for you to try.

It's Rough Waiting With VD

It's **R**ough	**R**enal failure
Waiting with	(**delayed** separation)
VD	**V**itamin **D**

Add 'Fanny' to the above to remind you of 'phosphate' – if you think it's necessary, as in 'It's Rough Waiting With VD, Fanny'.

Causes of **low phosphate** are high parathyroid hormone (PTH), low vitamin D and hypoventilation.

Lowly Phil Ate Dee's Breathless Parrot

Lowly **Ph**il ate	**Low Ph**osphate
Dee's	Vitamin **D** (low)
Breathless	Hypoventilation
Parro**t**	**PT**H (high)

Potassium – raised

What's behind raised potassium levels?

Too Much Pot Delayed Milo – Now Him Frigid

Too much pot	Hyperkalaemia
Delays	**Delay**ed separation of sample/difficult venesection
Milo	**Myelo**proliferative disorders
NOW	**NOW** take biochemistry samples, before any others!
Him	**H**aemolysis
Frigid	**Fridg**e (for storing blood)

Thyroid hormones

A **low serum free T4 level alone** could mean an underactive thyroid or pituitary gland failure. Therefore we need to look at the thyroid-stimulating hormone (TSH) level also. A **high TSH level alone** would confirm that the thyroid gland (not the pituitary gland) is responsible for the hypothyroidism. An underactive **'lazy' thyroid** gland gives us a **low T4 and a high TSH** – where the pituitary is 'flogging' the gland to get it to produce more thyroxine.

So think of:

Hitesh's Letter To Lazy Gland

Hite**sh**'s	**Hi TSH**
Letter **T**o	**L**ow **T**4
Lazy gland	**Lazy** thyroid **gland**

The usual cause of pituitary gland failure is tumour. So think:

Trish and Terry Fall in Pit

TriSH	Low **TSH**
and	**+**
Terry	**T**4
Fall in	**Falling** levels =
Pit	**Pit**uitary problem

To sum it all up:

Low T4 + **High** TSH = Lazy **Thyroid**
Low T4 + **Low** TSH = Failed **Pituitary**

SWOT BOX

A failing pituitary gland that is not producing TSH is not stimulating the thyroid to produce T4. Since the pituitary gland also regulates other glands (adrenals, gonads) as well as controlling growth and normal kidney function, failure means that the other glands may also be underactive.

Medicine is an art and attends to the nature of the (individual) patient and has principles of action and reason in each case
Plato (Symposium)

JOT BOX

MEDICAL SPECIALTIES

This chapter spans general medicine, cardiovascular and chest medicine, dermatology, endocrinology, gastroenterology, haematology, neurology, renal medicine and urology. As you read and learn about the subjects covered here you will be able to answer all the following, and more:

PRE-QUIZ

1 What does CREST stand for in CREST syndrome?
2 Can you list the features of acromegaly?
3 What are the X-ray features of Crohn's?
4 Which amino acids are not reabsorbed in cystinuria?
5 How would you manage diabetic ketoacidosis?
6 Can you name at least six causes of clubbing?
7 What are the ECG features of low potassium?
8 What are the six main types of exudate?
9 What are the risk factors for congenital dislocation of the hip?
10 Which pain fibres carry crude touch sensations?
11 Which nerve roots are affected if there is an absent biceps jerk reflex?
12 What are the main causes of mononeuritis multiplex?
13 What are the signs of a cerebellar lesion?

7.1 GENERAL MEDICINE AND PATHOLOGY

Bone metabolism

Osteoblasts build the bone and *osteoclasts* cut it away.

Blasts	**B**uild
Clasts	**C**ut away

Clubbing

Clubbing consists of loss of nail-bed angle, increased curvature of the nail (sideways and lengthways) and increased sponginess of the nail bed. The causes of clubbing are numerous. You can easily remember them when they are grouped like this:

The 8 Cs of Clubbing[1]

Carcinoma	Such as lung carcinoma or stomach carcinoma
Cardiac	Such as bacterial endocarditis or cyanotic congenital heart disease
Cervical rib	Causing neurovascular compression in the upper limb
Chest	Such as cystic fibrosis, empyema, bronchiectasis, tuberculosis (with extensive fibrosis), fibrosing alveolitis or abscess of lung
Circulation	Such as atrioventricular (AV) fistula in arm (kidney dialysis patients)
Cirrhosis	Of the liver (check for other signs of liver disease)
Colonic	Such as Crohn's, ulcerative colitis and coeliac disease
Congenital	

And here is an easy way to check for clubbing, known as the **'diamond' sign**. Put your thumbs together, back-to-back, with the thumbnails facing and touching each other. With normal nails you can see a thin diamond-shaped gap from the top of the knuckle to the top of the nail. This

1 This version is after A. Ala.

'diamond' is not seen with clubbing of the nails. If you draw this for yourself now, you are unlikely to forget it – the physical act will reinforce the memory.

SWOT BOX

Cervical ribs occur in 1% of the population, where embryological cervical elements form cervical ribs from C7. These may impinge on the subclavian artery and inferior trunk of the brachial plexus, resulting in neurovascular compression syndrome of the upper limb.

Neuroendocrine or **carcinoid tumours** produce a variety of different polypeptide hormones and products, especially serotonin (5-HT). Tumours are generally in the gastrointestinal tract and are often asymptomatic. Carcinoid syndrome (below) is usually associated with ileal carcinoids because hepatic decarboxylation is avoided.

Pseudo-clubbing occurs in thyroid disease.

And yet more on clubbing...

CLUB'D

C	**C**yanotic heart disease; Crohn's disease
L	**L**ung disease; liver disease
U	**U**lcerative colitis
B	**B**acterial endocarditis
D	**D**iarrhoea (chronic)

Crest syndrome

Here is a 'spatial' mnemonic for Crest syndrome, to remind you what it consists of. We can use a spatial mnemonics to learn this as there are five things we can easily link to the five digits of our own hand using exaggerated (and ridiculous) mental associations. Look at each digit in turn and picture as vividly as you can the following descriptions.

Symptom	Which digit	What to imagine as you look
Calcinosis	Thumb	Whoa! It's become completely calcified!
Raynaud's phenomenon	Index finger	It's bright blue and so cold!

Symptom	Which digit	What to imagine as you look
Oesophogeal dysmotility	Middle finger	Imagine sticking it down your throat like an endoscope
Sclerodactyly	Ring finger	Lots of tight rings that won't come off – so tight at the top of your finger that it's becoming tapered
Telangiectasia	Little finger	Hold it to your ear like a telephone (that's a 'substitute word' for telangiectasia)

> ## SWOT BOX
>
>
> **Calcinosis** is seen as palpable nodules in the hands due to calcific deposits in subcutaneous tissues.
>
> **Sclerodactyly** is tightening of the skin of the hand that leads to tapering of the fingers.
>
> **Telangiectasia** in Crest syndrome are multiple and large, and present on the hands.

For more on spatial mnemonics, see Section III.

Dupuytren's contracture

Dupuytren's is a fibrous contracture of the palmar fascia. You need to know the causes.

Alcoholic Doctors Fit a History of Trauma

Alcoholic	**Alcohol**
Doctors	**D**iabetes mellitus
Fit a	**Fit**s (as with epilepsy)
History of	**History** (family)
Trauma	**Trauma** (repeated, of the hand as in manual workers)

Alternative

You can add 'doped' to remind you of 'Dupuytren's' to make: Doped Alcoholic Doctors Fit a History of Trauma.

SWOT BOX

Baron Dupuytren (1777–1835) has a fascinating biography. He was kidnapped at the age of four by a wealthy lady (he was said to be a very attractive child) and later returned. He went to medical school in Paris and at age 18 was in charge of all the post mortems. We hear he was a very difficult person to get on with, perhaps due to this early trauma. He had early financial difficulties but ended up very wealthy, having built up a substantial practice. He suffered a stroke while lecturing in 1833 and died a few months later.

Exudates

An exudate is material that has escaped from blood vessels or tissues and is characterized by a high protein content. This mnemonic covers all the different types of exudate you need to know about.

Ham, sir? Remember Cats Prefer Fish

Ham	**H**aemorrhagic
Sir	**S**erous
Remember	**M**embranous
Cats	**C**atarrhal
Prefer	**P**urulent
Fish	**F**ibrinous

HLA-B27

Conditions associated with the **human leukocyte antigen** HLA-B27:

Hillbillies colliding sore ankles are irate

Hi**L**l**B**illies	**HL**A-**B**27
Colliding	**Col**itis
Sore	P**sor**iasis
Ankle**S**	**Ank**ylosing **S**pondylitis
are (**R**)	**R**eiter's
Irate	**Ir**itis (with the Reiter's)

Immunoglobulins

MARFANS[2]

M	(hyper) **M**obile joints
A	**A**uto dom 1:3000
R	**R**espiratory (bullae, bronchiectasis)
F	**F**ocus problems (dislocated lens, myopia, glaucoma)
A	**A**ortic aneurysm /dissection
N	**N**ervous system dural ectasia (= ballooning) seen on MRI; 65% get this
S	**S**keletal stature- arachnodatyl, tall, arm span > height

Rashes and fevers

The following anonymous chart is a guide to the day on which the rash typically appears after the prodrome – e.g. the rubella rash develops on the first day of the onset of fever/illness, and the scarlet fever rash appears on the second day. Note there is no rash appearing at day 6.

Really Sick People Must Take No Exercise

Really	**R**ubella	Day **1**
Sick	**S**carletina	Day **2**
People	small**P**ox	Day **3**
Must	**M**easles	Day **4**
Take	**T**yphoid fever	Day **5**
No	(**no**ne)	Day **6**
Exercise	**E**nteric fever	Day **7**

2 BHF Factfile November 2009, by KK and Suzy Jack, King's College Hospital, London.

Rheumatic fever

The five major (Jones's) criteria for **acute** rheumatic fever are carditis (40%), erythema marginatum (10–60%), subcutaneous nodules (10%), arthritis (migratory large-joint polyarthritis; 90%) and Sydenham's chorea (rapid, involuntary, purposeless and jerky movements, from Latin *chorea*; Greek *choreia*, meaning to dance). Some people use the mnemonic CHANCE, but even better than this is 'Arthur's Red Cardigan'.

Noodles and Curry On Arthur's Red Cardigan

Noodles and	**N**odules
Curry on	**C**horea
Arthur's	**A**rthritis
Red	**E**rythema
Cardigan	**C**arditis

SWOT BOX

The **acute** systemic illness is due to infection by a beta-haemolytic *Streptococcus*, usually between the ages of 5 and 15 years. The heart and joints are mainly affected. There may be myo-, endo- or pericarditis.

The minor criteria are **fe**ver, **a**rthralgia and **r**aised white cell count (**FeAR**). Confirmation of streptococcal infection and two major criteria are diagnostic (or one major and two minor).

If the attack is severe or occurs in early childhood or is recurrent, the disease may progress to chronic rheumatic heart disease (RHD). It is suggested that there is cross-reactivity between streptococcal and cardiac antigens. Chronic RHD is the largest global cause of heart disease, although it is less common in developed countries, probably due to the use of antibiotics (the streptococci are susceptible to penicillin).

Rheumatoid arthritis

This tells you the hand deformities in rheumatoid arthritis.

BUS'Z

B	**B**outonnière
U	**U**lnar deviation
S	**S**wan neck
Z	**Z** deformity (thumb)

It is also possible to see triggering of the finger (flexor tendon nodule) as well as erythema of the palms (which gives us BUSZ-TE).

Shock

These are the different types.

CASHED

C	**C**ardiac
A	**A**naphylactic
S	**S**eptic
H	**H**ypovolaemic
E	**E**ndocrine (e.g. Addison's)
D	**D**rugs (e.g. anaesthetics)

Syphilis

RAPID REVISION

This has already been covered (pages 58–9) but can you remember the stages and characteristics of syphilis? Do you recall that young lad from Bombay?

Vitamin D deficiency

Polly can help you remember the main features of this vitamin deficiency.

Polly Is Only A Shilling

Polly	**P**ernicious anaemia
Is	**I**ntrinsic factor (lack of)
Only	**O**nly confirmed if B12 deficiency is due to pernicious anaemia
A	**A**ntibodies vs parietal cells
Shilling	**Schilling** test

SWOT BOX

The **Schilling test** checks that the vitamin B12 deficiency is due to pernicious anaemia – which is correctable by giving **intrinsic factor**. In the test, parenteral radiolabelled B12 is given with oral B12. A 24-hour urine test demonstrates that oral B12 is not absorbed. The test is then with swallowed capsules of intrinsic factor – this corrects the deficiency due to pernicious anaemia *only*.

JOT BOX

7.2 CARDIOLOGY

PRE-QUIZ

1 What is the incidence of atrial fibrillation in people in their eighties? And in their fifties?
2 Can you list the causes of central cyanosis?
3 What are the features associated with coarctation of the aorta?
4 What are the main features of aortic stenosis?

Aortic stenosis

For the main features, remember:

Middle-Aged Men Force Thrills Slowly

Middle-aged **M**en	**Mid**-systolic **M**urmur
Force	**Force**ful apex beat
Thrills	systolic **Thrill** (at base of heart)
Slowly	**Slow** rising pulse

Atrial fibrillation

The three types of atrial fibrillation (AF) can be classified as PERsistent, PARoxysmal or PERManent – that is, three Ps. Yet despite so many Ps, atrial fibrillation is characterized by a lack of P waves on the ECG! Which gives us:

3 Ps – But no 'p' on ECG!

Alternative

PERcy's PARrot's PERM, or just PPP.

SWOT BOX

Incidence of AF[3,4]

- **0.5**% at **5**0–59 years (Point five per cent of people in their fifties)
- **8.8**% at **8**0–**8**9 years of age (8.8 per cent of people aged 88)
- Paroxysmal = Self-resolving, duration < 48 hours
- Persistent = Duration > 48 hours. May or may not be self-terminating
- Permanent = > Cardioversion not feasible or failed

Causes of AF

Include: hypertension; heart disease (including valve disease, congenital heart disease, sick sinus syndrome); thyrotoxicosis; drugs (e.g. caffeine, nicotine, ethanol); pulmonary diseases; sleep apnoea; inflammation and infection.

Bundle branch block classics

What happens to the shape of the ECG when there is a bundle branch block?

With a **right branch block** there is an M-shaped wave in V1, and sometimes a W-shaped wave in V6. To remember this, think of a marrow:

MARROW

Ma	V1
RRo	(**right** bundle branch block)
W	V6

With a **left branch block** you get a W-shaped complex in V1 and occasionally an M-shaped complex in V6. Thanks to William we get:

WILLIAM

Wi	V1
LLia	(**left** bundle branch block)
M	V6

3 Kannel WB, Abbott RD, Savage DD, McNamara PM (1982) Epidemiologic features of chronic atrial fibrillation: the Framingham study. *N Engl J Med* 306(17):1018–22.
4 Lip GYH, Li Saw Hee FL (2001) Paroxysmal atrial fibrillation. *QJM* 94(12):665–78.

Cardiac troponins

There are three types of troponins – C, T and I. Troponins C and I are the cardiac ones. They are very sensitive indicators of cardiac damage, but they are not too specific, so this rule of Cs will help you to know the other six major causes of raised cardiac troponins.

The C Rule

Cardiac arrest	myocardial infarction
Cardiac failure	severe heart failure
Cocaine	causes coronary artery spasm
Carditis	myocarditis
Car accident	or some other trauma
Chest	pulmonary emboli

SWOT BOX

Cardiac troponins are released from striated muscles cells within 12 hours of cardiac damage. They are present for several days after the event.

Central cyanosis

The causes of central cyanosis are made quite memorable with this mnemonic.

Tense Fresher's Cope Emphasizing Arty 'Pnemonics'!

Tense	**T**ension pneumothorax
Fresher's	**F**ibrosing alveolitis
Cope	**COP**D
Emphasizing	**Emph**ysema
Arty	**A**sthma
Pnemonics!	**Pneumon**ia

Coarctation of the aorta

The natural history of aortic coarctation involves hypertension, heart failure, aortic aneurysm rupture, endocarditis, and aortic valve disease (regurgitation, stenosis, biscuspid valves). To remind yourself of these important features you could think of:

Hyperactive Avril Oughta Fail Endo

Hyperactive	Hypertension
AVRil	**A**ortic **V**alve disease (including **R**egurgitation, **AVR**)
Oughta	**Aorta** (rhymes) (aneurysm rupture)
Fail	heart **Fail**ure
Endo	**Endo**carditis

Congestive cardiac failure

Left ventricular failure (LVF) manifests as acute difficulty in breathing, while right ventricular failure (RVF) tends to cause swellings in peripheral areas and is particularly evident in the lower limbs. Think:

LVF affects the **L**ungs

RVF affects the **R**est (leading to fluid overload)

Here is a useful way to remember the signs of **fluid overload** caused by right ventricular failure:

Fat Ella Jumps and Gallops Over Livid Plums

Fat	**F**atigue
Ella **J**umps and	**E**levated **J**VP
Gallops	**G**allop rhythm – S3 heart sound
Over	**O**edema
Livid	**Liv**er enlarged
Plums	**Pl**eural effusion

ECG leads

Connecting up the ECG leads is easy when you think of some traffic lights – they have to be broken ones so they end in 'black'. Start *clockwise* from the right side of the patient:

Traffic lights

Red	**Right** arm
Yellow	Left arm
Green	Left leg
Black	Right leg

Alternative

Read Your Good Book, *or* Ride Your Green Bike.

Why don't you reinforce this by sketching a DaVinci-style body on a clock face with all four limbs stretching out to the edge of the clock?

Heart rate is determined from the big squares on the ECG trace like this:

Number of big squares	Heart rate (beats per minute)
1	300
2	150
3	100
4	75
5	60
6	50

Endocarditis

The main features of endocarditis are given by:

Splendid Feverish Vegetarians Enjoy Clubbing Till a.m.

Splendid	**Splen**omegaly
Feverish	**Fever** (> 1 week, > 38.5°C)
Vegetarians	**Veget**ations (on echo)
Enjoy	**E**mboli (come off the vegetations)
Clubbing	**Clubbing**
Till	**T**ricuspid valve (in IV drug abusers)
a.m.	**A**ortic and **M**itral valves (usually affected)

The infecting organisms in endocarditis are shown here.

Grannie Enjoys Straps and Staples

Grannie	**Gra**m **n**egative bacteria
Enjoys	**En**terococci
Straps and	**Strep**tococci
Staples	**Stap**hylococci

Hypertension

The causes of hypertension are made far more memorable with this quick reminder.

CREEEP

C	**C**oarctation of the aorta
R	**R**enal
E	**E**ndocrine
E	**E**clampsia
E	**E**ssential (i.e. unknown cause – the majority)
P	**P**ill or **P**haeocromocytoma

Left atrial enlargement (P mitrale)

The ECG of this condition shows a bifid P wave (of duration 0.12 seconds or more). The two peaks are due to delayed response from the enlarged left atrium. The first peak is from the right atrium, and the second is from the left. In P mitrale, therefore, the trace looks like a letter 'm', so remember:

P **m**itrale looks like letter '**m**'   (**m** for **m**itrale)

Draw this quickly to reinforce the image in your head.

Lipoproteins

Here's how to distinguish between good and bad lipoproteins. Very-low-density lipoproteins (VLDLs) carry triglycerides from hepatic to peripheral and other cells, where they are stored and later used for metabolism. High-density lipoproteins (HDLs) carry cholesterol away from the peripheral cells to the liver for excretion. Therefore, you can think of them as:

H (for **H**DL) are **H**eroes
V (for **V**LDL) are **V**illains

Mitral stenosis

According to Rubenstein and Wayne,[5] the development of pulmonary hypertension in mitral stenosis is indicated by APRIL.

5 Rubenstein D, Wayne D (2002) *Lecture Notes in Clinical Medicine*. Edinburgh: Blackwells.

APRIL

A	**A** dominant 'a' wave of the jugular venous pulse (unless in atrial fibrillation)
P	**P**ulmonary valve (second sound is loud)
R	**R**ight ventricular hypertrophy
I	**I**ncompetence (pulmonary – rare)
L	**L**ow peripheral arterial pulse volume

Murmurs and heart sounds

RAPID REVISION

Before we cover systolic and diastolic murmurs, we need a quick reminder about **heart sounds**. On the front cover we learn about the Mighty Ape, as a convenient way to relate the mitral (M) and tricuspid (T) components and aortic (A) and pulmonary (P) valve closures.

Diastolic murmurs can be summed up by DAIMS.

DAIMS

D	**D**iastolic
AI	**A**ortic **I**ncompetence
MS	**M**itral **S**tenosis

SWOT BOX

So on the flip side, you can also work out that systolic murmurs are the opposite, i.e. aortic stenosis and mitral incompetence.

Remember **more systolic murmurs** using this phrase:

As Innocent Mr Terry Passes VD

AS	**A**ortic **S**tenosis
Innocent	**Innocent** murmur
MR	**M**itral **R**egurgitation (**MR**)
TeRry	**T**ricuspid **R**egurgitation (**TR**)
PASSes	**P**ulmon**A**ry **S**tenosi**S**
VD	**V**entricular septal **D**efect

Pericarditis

In pericarditis the ECG trace characteristically shows a 'saddle-shaped', raised ST segment in most leads. You:

Park Your **C**ar [**PeriC**arditis] before you **S**i**T** in a saddle

As awful as this statement is, you will now always remember the ST saddle shape on the ECG in pericarditis... groan!

Plasma potassium – low

When plasma potassium drops, the shape of the ECG changes, the height of the T wave becomes flattened. Thus, you should remember:

No Pot No Tea!

On the flip side, high K causes peaked T waves:

Big Pot High Tea!

Prevention of heart disease

Secondary prevention of heart disease after myocardial infarct includes the following:

ACE–ABC

ACE	**ACE** inhibitors
A	**A**ntiplatelets
B	**B**eta blocker
C	**C**alcium-channel blocker

Raynaud's phenomenon

Raynaud's manifests as intermittent ischaemia of the fingers and toes with severe pallor, cyanosis, pain and numbness. WBC gives the colour changes observed in the extremities in Raynaud's, in order.

Raynaud's WBC

White	Arteriolar spasm
Blue	Dilated capillaries (skin feels cold, numb)
Crimson red	Reactive hyperaemia (as the vasospasm relaxes)

SWOT BOX

Raynaud was a French physician (1834–1881). His 'phenomenon' was the subject of his thesis. Raynaud's is aggravated by cold or emotional stimuli and relieved by heat, and is secondary to some other abnormality, such as systemic lupus erythematosus (SLE), scleroderma, cervical rib, trauma from vibrating tools, or drugs such as beta blockers, ergotamine and oral oestrogens. When the cause is primary, familial or idiopathic, it is called Raynaud's disease. The latter is more common in women.

Raynaud's **D**isease we **D**on't know
Phenomenon has a **P**athological cause

Some of the causes are listed in Chapter 9, Surgical Specialties, under the mnemonic: My Servant's Vibrator's So Cold, Ergo Dame's Thighs Are Nervous.

Rheumatic fever

RAPID REVISION

You may remember the five major criteria (Jones's criteria) for **acute rheumatic fever**, which are carditis, erythema marginatum, subcutaneous nodules, arthritis and Sydenham's chorea, as specified by the mnemonic 'Noodles and Curry on Arthur's Red Cardigan' (see p. 74).

Volume depletion

The signs of depletion are conveniently explained by one word – DEPLETE.

DEPLETE

D	**D**ry mucous membranes
E	**E**xtremities are cold
P	**P**ulse faint (postural hypotension)
L	**L**oss of weight
E	**E**lectrolytes abnormal
T	**T**achycardia
E	**E**lasticity of skin (turgor) is reduced

7.3 CHEST MEDICINE

Haemoptysis

These are the major causes.

Cancel new tablets – bring crone blood

Cancel	**C**ancer
New	**Pn**eumonia
Tablets	**T**uberculosis
Bring	**B**ronchiectasis
Crone	**C**hronic bronchitis
Blood	**B**lood clot (pulmonary embolism)

Pleuritic pain

How can you learn all the causes of pleuritic pain? Try this:

Concert News: Fresher Slips Sucking Paul's Shiny Muscular Pen

Concert	**C**ancer
News	**Pn**eumonia
Fresher	**F**racture
Slips	**S**lipped disc (neuropathic pain)
Sucking	**C**oxsackie virus (Bornholm's)
Paul's	**P**leurisy
Shiny	**Sh**ingles
Muscular	**M**usculoskeletal injury
PEn	**P**ulmonary **E**mbolus

Respiratory failure

Here are some tips for remembering the features of types 1 and 2 respiratory failure. In both types, oxygen is lost but we measure parameters of oxygen and carbon dioxide. In type 1, oxygen is low (only one parameter is affected). In type 2, both carbon dioxide and oxygen are affected.

Type	Parameters affected[6]
1	**1** (oxygen)
2	**2** (oxygen and carbon dioxide)

Stridor and wheeze

Stridor is a harsh, grating and frequently high-pitched breath sound; it is almost always inspiratory, produced by upper respiratory obstruction (such as in croup). **Wheezes** are polyphonic, high-pitched sounds, usually caused by intrapulmonary airways obstruction. They are usually expiratory sounds. How do you remember the difference? Simple:

St**I**dor	In**SpI**ratory
Wh**EE**z**E**	**E**xpiratory....

SWOT BOX

The causes of stridor include laryngotracheobronchitis or croup (mainly parainfluenza type III virus), foreign bodies, *Haemophilus influenzae* type B infection, epiglottitis (or 'supraglottitis'), upper respiratory inflammation (from corrosive/hot/irritant fumes and gases), laryngomalacia (congenital floppy larynx), congenital vascular ring, retropharyngeal abscess, post- intubation, *Corynebacterium diphtheriae* infection (diphtheria), angioedema and tetany and mediastinal masses.

Tuberculosis

See more about TB treatment in Chapter 4, Pharmacology, and Chapter 5, Microbiology and infectious diseases.

JOT BOX

6 Dr Shahid Khan, Consultant Hepatologist, St Mary's Hospital, London.

7.4 DERMATOLOGY

Epiloia (tuberous sclerosis)

This is rare (except in textbooks). It is autosomal dominant disorder of the skin and central nervous system, diagnosed in childhood. Important clinical features include **shagreen patches**, **subungual fibromas** (smooth, pinkish projections which grow from the nail base), **retinal phakomas** (white streaks along the fundal vessels – epiloia is often classed as a phacomatosis), **adenoma sebaceum** (pinkish papules on facial skin which can be confused with acne) and **ash-leaf macules** (elongated or ovoid hypopigmented macules). It is a cause of learning difficulty. This mnemonic is suitably rude.

So there was that ol' **shagger** from Bourneville

Who bit off his **fibromas**, **subungual**

'Oh **phakoma**!' he cried

'These **adenomas** won't hide –

and all these **ash-leaves** just look like a jungle!'

SWOT BOX

This is also known as Bourneville's disease after a French neurologist.

Hair cycle

The phases of the hair's growth cycle are given by the acronym ACT.

ACT

Anagen   (longest phase)

Catagen

Telogen   (resting phase)

Hair loss occurring about 3 months after pregnancy or major illness is considered as telogen-phase hair loss.

Kaposi's sarcoma

KAPOSI reminds you what to look out for:

KAPOSI

K	**C**onjunctivitis
A	**A**IDS-defining illness (1993 classification)
P	**P**alate lesions
O	**O**ther sites (e.g. lungs and lymph nodes)
S	**S**kin
I	**I**ndigestion (the GI tract is affected)

Keratoacanthoma

Keratoacanthoma looks like a *volcano* because of a central keratin plug which often comes off. To remember this, remember the condition as:

Krakatoa – Acanthoma!

> ## SWOT BOX
>
> Keratoacanthoma is an overgrowth of pilosebaceous glands (hair follicle cells) with potential for malignancy, although it is self-limiting in most cases. It is often mistaken for a squamous cell carcinoma.

Papules

Papules are small and elevated skin lesions (unlike maculae). So remember:

Papules are **P**alpable

Pemphigus vs pemphigoid

Is there an easy way to remember the difference between them? You bet!

Pemphigu**S**	**S**uperficial
Pemphigoi**D**	**D**eep

SWOT BOX

Pemphigus is a group of skin diseases with vesicles and bullae, acantholysis on histology and antiepidermal autoantibodies.

Pemphigoid has cleft formation at the dermoepidermal junction, while immunofluorescence reveals complement and IgG deposits at the level of the lamina lucida of the basement membrane. Yes, you've read it before.

Ultraviolet A vs B

UVA rays penetrate through the epidermis better than UVB rays, so they have different effects in general.

UV**A**   **A**geing (of the skin, wrinkles)
UV**B**   **B**urning, **B**rowning and **B**lindness (cataracts)

Xerostoma

Xerostoma means 'mouth dryness'. So think about this condition as xerosaliva – zero saliva.

Zero saliva makes your mouth dry!

JOT BOX

7.5 ENDOCRINOLOGY

Acromegaly

Amazingly, each of the first ten letters of the alphabet describes one or more features of acromegaly.

A-B-C-D-E-F-G-H-I-J

A	**A**rthropathy
B	**B**ig boggy hands
C	**C**arpal tunnel syndrome
D	**D**iabetes
E	**E**nlarged tongue, heart and throat
F	**F**ields (bitemporal hemianopia)
G	**G**ynaecomastia, **G**alactorrhoea and **G**reasy skin
H	**H**ypertension (20–50%)
I	**I**ncreasing size (of shoes, hat, gloves, dentures, rings)
J	**J**aw enlargement and prognathism

Anterior pituitary hormones

The six anterior pituitary hormones are thyroid-stimulating hormone (TSH), growth hormone (GH), the gonadotrophins (luteinizing hormone (LH) and follicle-stimulating hormone (FSH)), prolactin and adrenocorticotrophic hormone (ACTH).

Those Giant Gonads Prolong the Action

Those	**T**SH
Giant	**G**H
Gonads	LH/FSH
Prolong the	**P**rolactin
Action	**A**CTH

Carcinoid syndrome

It's hard to believe, but every letter of the word carcinoid describes one of its features!

CARCINOID

C	**C**yanosis
A	**A**sthma
R	**R**ubor
C	**C**or pulmonale
I	**I**ncompetent tricuspid/pulmonary valve
N	**N**oisy abdomen
O	**O**edema
I	**I**ndoles in stools
D	**D**iarrhoea

SWOT BOX

Carcinoid tumours are neuroendocrine in origin and produce a variety of different polypeptide hormones and products, especially serotonin (5-HT). Tumours are generally in the gastrointestinal tract and are often asymptomatic.

Carcinoid syndrome is usually associated with ileal carcinoids because hepatic decarboxylation is avoided.

Cushing's – causes

Important causes of Cushing's are easily remembered courtesy of Adrienne's stereo:

Adrienne's Top ACT – Put Stereo On!

Adrienne's	**Adr**enal tumour
Top ACT	ec**TOP**ic **ACT**H
Put	**P**ituitary adenoma
Stereo on	**Ster**oids

Alternative

Cushion [Cushing's] Put On Top Of Adrienne's Stereo

Cushing's vs Addison's

Students often confuse these two endocrine conditions. To clarify think:

ADDison's due to **AD**renal **D**amage

(Think **ADD** due to **AD-D**)

Cushing's caused by too much **C**ortisol

Diabetic ketoacidosis

I am grateful to Dr R. Clarke of Barnet General Hospital for this suggested scheme pertaining to the emergency management of diabetic ketoacidosis (DKA).

PANICS

P	**P**otassium
A	**A**spirate stomach (nasogastric tube)
N	**N**ormal saline
I	**I**nsulin infusion
C	**C**ultures (midstream urine, blood)/catheterize
S	**S**ubcutaneous heparin

Diabetes mellitus

Complications of diabetes mellitus are indicated by KNIVES.

KNIVES

K	**K**idney	Glomerular sclerosis; uraemia; hypertension; nephrotic syndrome; renal papillary necrosis; atherosclerosis of renal vessels; effects of hypertension
N	**N**euromuscular	Peripheral neuropathy; mononeuritis (see p. 109) autonomic neuropathy; diabetic amyotrophy

I	Infective	Urinary tract, skin and soft tissue infection; tuberculosis; moniliasis; pyelonephritis
V	Vascular	Large vessel → ischaemic heart disease Small vessel → microangiopathy
E	Eye	Cataracts; background proliferative and pre-proliferative retinopathy; microaneurysms; maculopathy; fibrosis; retinal detachment; photocoagulation spots of retinal burns
S	Skin	Lipoatrophy and insulin sensitivity at injection site; necrobiosis lipoidica; granuloma annulare

Diffuse goitre

These are the causes of diffuse goitre.[7]

Limp Simon's Silent Grave is Stashed with Hash

Limp	Lymphoma
Simon's	Simple non-toxic goitre
Silent	Silent thyroiditis (painless)
Grave is	Grave's
Stashed with	Subacute thyroiditis
Hash	Hashimoto's

Here is another useful version.[8]

Simple Substances Like Hash Get You Sex

Simple	Simple non-toxic goitre
Substances	Subacute thyroiditis
Like	Lymphoma

---

7 Contributed by Sana Haroon BSc (2007).
8 Contributed by Dr Majeed Mussalam BSc (2007).

Hash	**Hash**imoto's
Get you	**G**rave's
Sex	**S**ilent thyroiditis

Parathyroid glands

There are four interesting facts about the parathyroid glands.

All 4s

4 glands
4th (and 3rd) branchial arch is where they arise
40 mg in weight
40 mm in diameter

Phaeochromocytoma

This is a usually benign, well-encapsulated lobular tumour of chromaffin cells in the adrenal medulla. It mainly presents as raised blood pressure (see CREEEP on p. 82). Attacks also cause palpitations, sweating, tremor and nausea.

10 per cent rule

10% are multiple
10% are malignant
10% are adrenal bilateral
10% are extra-adrenal
10% are familial
10% are in children[9]

The 10% ACME rule has its place too:

10% ACME

10% are:

A	**A**drenal (bilateral)
C	**C**hildren
M	**M**alignant
E	**E**xtra-adrenal

9 Figures from *Update* (10/6/1998) p. 1130.

Secondary hyperparathyroidism

Primary hyperparathyroidism accounts for 30% of cases of raised calcium levels (remember: bones, stones, moans and abdominal groans). But in **secondary hyperparathyroidism** the calcium is lowered. This is because chronically low plasma calcium levels are the cause of the compensatory increase in PTH secretion. After reading Section III, try coming back to make a 'link' mnemonic for these 10 Cs.

The 10 Cs of secondary hyperparathyroidism

Calcium down
Cramps
Carpopedal spasms
Chvostek's sign
Convulsions
Cataracts
Cavities (dental)
Crazy (change in mental state)
Cardiac arrhythmias
Cranial pressure rises

Solitary thyroid nodules

To remember the causes, remember about the heroin, acid, hash and coke.

Sold Students Heroin, Acid, Hash 'n' Coke

Sold	**S**olitary
Students	**C**ysts
Heroin	**H**aemorrhage
Acid	**A**denoma
Hash	**Hash**imoto's
'n'	big **N**odule
Coke	**C**arcinoma

7.6 GASTROENTEROLOGY

Cirrhosis

The complications of cirrhosis are listed under PAPAH.

PAPAH

P	**P**ortal hypertension
A	**A**scites
P	**P**ortosystemic encephalopathy
A	**A**cute renal failure
H	**H**epatocellular carcinoma

Gastrointestinal bleeding

The causes of bleeding of the upper gastrointestinal tract are given by VARICES. There are idiopathic causes in 2–4% of cases.

V	**V**arices
A	**A**lcohol and drugs
R	**R**upture (Mallory–Weiss)
I	**I**diopathic (in 2–4%)
C	**C**arcinoma
E	o**E**sophagitis or gastric **E**rosion
S	**S**tomach (gastric ulcer or duodenal ulcer)

Gum hypertrophy

A good way to remember the causes:

Look! Funny Crowns!

Look	**L**eukaemia
Funny	**Ph**enytoin
Crowns	**C**rohn's or **C**iclosporin

Hepatitis B

The risk groups for hepatitis B are given by the 6 Hs.[10]

The 6 Hs of hepatitis B

Health workers (have you had your jabs yet?)
Heroin (or other intravenous drug abusers)
Haemophiliacs
Homosexuals
Haemodialysis
Homes (people in institutions)

Hepatomegaly

Hepatomegaly has five main causes as described here.

Hippies Sell Space In Congested Bedsit

Hippies	**Hep**atomegaly is caused by:
Sell	**Cell**ular proliferation
Space	**Space**-occupying lesions
In	**In**filtration
Congested	**Congest**ion
BedSi**T**	**B**il**E D**uct ob**ST**ruction

Inflammatory bowel disease

Treatment of inflammatory bowel disease (IBD) includes a number of drugs.

Curt flogs Cyndi's Meaty Ass

Curt	**C**orticosteroids
Flogs	**Fl**agyl (metronidazole)
Cyndi's	**C**iclosporins
Meaty	**M**ethotrexate
Ass	**A**zathioprine and **A**minosalicylates (5-ASA)

---

10 Collier JAB, Longmore M, Brinsden M (1999) *Oxford Handbook of Clinical Specialties*, 5th edn. Oxford: Oxford University Press.

You may prefer this reminder:

And as Curt Met Cindy

And **A**s	**A**zathioprine and **A**minosalicylates (5-ASA)
Curt	**C**orticosteroids
Met	**Met**hotrexate and **Met**ronidazole
Cindy	**C**iclosporins

Pancreatitis

Causes of pancreatitis are given by this very well-known mnemonic.

GET SMASH'D

G	**G**allstones
E	**E**thanol
T	**T**rauma
S	**S**teroids
M	**M**umps
A	**A**utoimmune disease
S	**S**corpion bites
H	**H**yperlipidaemia
D	**D**rugs

And the investigations of pancreatitis are encapsulated here:

O, Claw Gut

O	**O**xygen (blood gases)
C	**C**alcium
L	**L**actate dehydrogenase
A	**A**mylase
W	**W**hite cell count
G	**G**lucose
U	**U**rea
T	**T**ransaminase

Ulcerative colitis

The features of a severe attack of ulcerative colitis often involve low serum albumin (< 30 g/litre), fever (> 37.5°C), anaemia (Hb < 10 g%), tachycardia, high erythrocyte sedimentation rate (ESR > 30 mm/hour) and bloody diarrhoea. A useful mnemonic is given here.

SHITER

S	**S**erum albumin ↓
H	**H**igh fever
I	**I**ron deficiency (anaemia)
T	**T**achycardia
E	**E**SR ↑
R	**R**ed (blood) in diarrhoea

JOT BOX

7.7 HAEMATOLOGY

Anaemia

There are FIVE ways to treat anaemia.[11]

FIVE

F	**F**olate
I	**I**ron
V	**V**itamin B12
E	**E**rythropoietin

Direct Coombs test

This tests for haemolytic anaemia with an immune cause.

HICCUP

H	**H**aemolytic anaemia of...
I	**I**mmunological...
C	**C**ause →
C	**C**oombs test is...
U	**U**sually...
P	**P**ositive

Favism (G6PD deficiency)

To remember that favism (G6PD deficiency) is associated with Heinz bodies in the red blood cell (on blood film or methyl violet stain), imagine a tin of Heinz 'Fava' Beans.

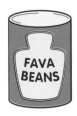

FAVA BEANS

---

11 From Sarah Gates, St Andrews University, 2005.

SWOT BOX

The full name of the enzyme G6PD is **glucose-6-phosphate dehydrogenase**. It is involved in the **hexose monophosphate shunt** involved in glutathione reduction. It is essential for protecting red cell membranes from oxidative crises. If the cell is lacking in reduced glutathione, nothing protects the haemoglobin from being oxidized, precipitating rapid anaemia with jaundice.

The oxidized haemoglobin precipitates within the cell to form **Heinz bodies**, which stick to the membrane and make it more rigid.

Splenic macrophages lyse the inclusion-bearing cells. This can happen with fava beans (*Vicia faba*), illness, antimalarial drugs or other drugs such as sulfonamides.

Haemophilias A and B

Haemophilia A is due to lack of factor 8 and haemophilia B is due to lack of factor 9. Think of:

Factor **8**   **A**ight (rather than Eight)
Factor **q**   **b** (upside down)

Lymphadenopathy

Causes of lymph node enlargement include sarcoid, syphilis, metastatic disease (e.g. lympho- and reticulosarcomas), primary reticuloses, lymphogranuloma, glandular fever and TB.

Sarcastic Sybil Met Trouble in Ridiculing Grannie's Gift

Sarcastic   **Sarc**oid
Sybil   **Sy**philis
Met   **Met**astatic disease
TrouBle   **TuB**erculosis
In   **N**on-specific
Ridiculing   **R**eticuloses
Grannie's   lympho**GRAN**uloma
GiFt   **G**landular **F**ever

MCV – causes of raised

Remember the causes of raised MCV using this:

Between Infections My Laura Felt Bloody Happy

Between	**B**12 (low)
Infections	**Infections**
My	**M**arrow/myelodysplasias
Laura	**L**iver disease/alcohol abuse
Felt	**F**olate (low)
Bloody	**Blood** loss
Happy	**H**ypothyroidism

Sickle cell and glutamine

The sickle cell beta-globin gene causes valine to be replaced by glutamine at position 6. So think of:

Glute's in position sex

| **Glut**e's in | **Glut**amine |
| Position **sex** | Position **six** |

Now, you already know that the homozygous state of the haemoglobin (Hb) structure in this condition is designated *HbSS*, and heterozygous as *HbAS*. So let's link *HbAS* to facts we need to learn:

HbAS

H	**H**ypoxia, haemolytic crises
b	**B**eta chain affected
A	**A**plastic crises, acute sequestration crises
S	**S**ixth position of Hb beta chain
	Symptoms start at age **S**ix months (fetal Hb present before 6 months)
	Sodium metabisulfite test (induces **S**ickling *in vitro*)

Unconjugated bilirubin

RAPID REVISION

Here's a quick question for you. What are the causes of unconjugated bilirubin? If you don't know them yet, then check p. 64 for a cool mnemonic!

7.8 NEUROLOGY

> *More brain, O Lord, more brain!*
> George Meredith

Bell's palsy

It is absolutely crucial that you can distinguish between a Bell's palsy and a central lesion (e.g. ischaemic stroke – which requires urgent management). In Bell's palsy, *both* the upper and the lower parts of the face are affected (i.e. both upper and lower face paralyses).

Remember:

Bell's affects **B**oth

SWOT BOX

The facial nerves originate in the motor cortex, and supply the muscles of facial expression. But on their way through the brainstem (pons), some fibres cross over to join the opposite (contralateral) facial nerve – hence the muscles of the **upper** part of the face have a **bilateral** nerve supply. The **lower** face/mouth has a nerve supply from the **contralateral** hemisphere ONLY.

An upper-motor neuron lesion (e.g. stroke) causes contralateral paralysis of the **lower** face/mouth. The patient is **able to close their eyes, raise their eyebrows and wrinkle their forehead** (because they have the motor input from the opposite cortex). With Bell's palsy, ipsilateral motor supply to BOTH upper and lower face is affected.

Patients struggle to close their eyelid (need an eye patch and eye drops) and have a droopy mouth, i.e. in **B**ell's palsy **b**oth upper face and lower face are affected.

Cerebellar signs

This is a common subject in exams. It is definitely worth knowing the following mnemonic well.[12]

---

12 From Dr Robert Clarke (2004–2007) *Medicine for Finals*. Dr Clarke's Revision Courses in Association with the BMA.

DANISH

D	**D**ysdiadochokinesia
A	**A**taxia
N	**N**ystagmus
I	**I**ntention tremor (approx. 3 Hz)
S	**S**peech (**S**canning/**S**taccato)
H	**H**ypotonia

SWOT BOX

Cerebellar signs are ipsilateral to a lesion.

Dysdiadochokinesia is impairment in ability to perform rapidly alternating movements such as sequential supination and pronation.

Ataxia (Greek, *taxis* = order; *a* = negative) is lack of muscular coordination, and it leads to an abnormal gait; the patient often staggers and walks with a broad-based gait for stability, tending to fall in the direction of the side of the lesion.

Cerebellar nystagmus is usually horizontal (ask the patient to look laterally); the 'finger–nose' test shows the 'past-pointing' effect of the **intention tremor**, whereby on being asked to touch their nose, the patient misses and hits their cheek). Note that tremor is not affected by closing the eyes and occurs during a movement – not at rest (unlike Parkinson's disease).

Speech is often affected (dysarthria) and sometimes described as 'slurred and explosive'.

The **muscles** are often **hypotonic** but may be hypertonic also, which (of course) aggravates the ataxia.

Claw hand

There are many causes of claw hand which this mnemonic may help you to remember.

Um...VW Brake-Pads Made In Romania Suck

UM	**U**lnar and **M**edian nerve palsy
VW	**V**olkmann's contracture (ischaemia)

Brake-**P**ads	**B**rachial **P**lexus lesion of...
Made	**M**edial cord
In	**I**njury
Romania	**R**heumatoid arthritis
SuCk	**S**pinal **C**ord lesion

Among the injuries that cause claw hand are scarring, trauma and burns. The spinal cord lesions include polio, syringomyelia and lateral amyotrophic sclerosis (remember these as *Pull Strings Laterally, Amy*).

Pull Strings Laterally, Amy

Pull	**P**olio
Strings	**S**yringomelia
Laterally	**Lateral**
Amy	**Amy**otrophic sclerosis

Coma

You can distinguish between pontine and cerebral causes of coma by the direction of deviation of the eyes.

Pontine lesions	Eyes **P**oint to **P**aralysed limbs
Cerebral lesion	Eyes **S**tare at **S**atisfactory limbs

> ## SWOT BOX
>
> The eyes may deviate away from the midline due to cerebral hemisphere lesions where they 'look' towards the side of the lesion (i.e. towards the normal limbs). With pontine lesions, this generally occurs in the opposite direction, so the eyes deviate away from the side of the lesion towards the affected limbs.

Epileptic seizures

This anonymous and ancient rhyme (from the days when the word 'fit' was widely used) neatly sums up the features of epileptic seizures.

The aura, the cry, the fall, the fit
The tonus, the clonus, the pee and the shit
Describes an epileptic fit

Obviously, this describes the features of a *tonic* (spasm) and *clonic* (jerking) seizure. It is useful for determining whether or not the fit was epileptiform. You do, of course, need to be aware of the wide variety of clinical patterns of epilepsy – including altered motor and sensory phenomena, altered consciousness and sometimes odd behaviour.

See more on treatment of epilepsy on p. 51.

Examination

Here is a simple mnemonic for remembering what to include in a standard neurological examination.[13]

That Physician Really Is So Cool

That	**T**one
Physician	**P**ower
Really	**R**eflexes
Is	**I**nspection
So	**S**ensation
Cool	**C**oordination/orientation

Friedreich's ataxia

These are the main features and associations.

French Taxi Cars ARe Scarce, Babe

FRench	**FR**iedreich
TAXI	a**TAXI**a
CARs	**CAR**diomyopathy
ARe	**A**utosomal **R**ecessive
SCarce	**SC**oliosis
BABe	**BAB**inski sign (positive: also have high arched plantars)

Note that the Babinski sign is present in patients with Friedreich's ataxia. They will also have high-arched plantars.

13 Attributed to Dr Sheetle Shah, Croydon.

Gait abnormalities

The causes of abnormal gait are numerous, as summarized here.

All Patients Spending Cash See Proper Doctors[14]

All	**A**praxia/ataxia
Patients	**P**arkinsonism
Spending	**S**pasticity
Cash	**C**erebellar ataxia
See	**S**ensory deficit
Proper	**P**roximal myopathy
Doctors	**D**istal myopathy

Gerstmann syndrome

This syndrome is a combination of four symptoms and can be remembered quite easily.

A-ALF

A	**A**graphia
A	**A**calculia
L	**L**eft–right disorientation
F	**F**inger agnosia

14 With thanks to Stuart McCorkel, SGMMS 1990.

SWOT BOX

Gerstmann's is due to a lesion in the angular gyrus of the dominant hemisphere. *Agraphia* means the inability to write. *Acalculia* is similar but relates to the ability to perform simple arithmetic calculations. *Agnosia* is the loss of recognition of sensory stimuli. The syndrome is named after Josef Gerstmann, a Viennese neurologist (1887–1969).

Mononeuritis multiplex

SCALD will remind you of causes of this disease.

SCALD

S	**S**arcoid
C	**C**arcinoma
A	**A**rteritis
L	**L**eprosy
D	**D**iabetes

Myotonic dystrophy

Popular in exams, this is a rare condition affecting only 5 in 10 000, which often becomes more severe in successive generations. Use the first nine letters of the alphabet to help you with some of the main features.

A-B-C-D-E-F-G-H-I

A	**A**trophy or if autosomal dominant
B	**B**aldness (frontal, in males)
C	**C**ataracts or if **C**hromosome 9 affected
D	**D**roopy eyes or **D**ysphagia or **D**iabetes (if end organs do not respond to insulin)
E-F	**E**xpressionless **F**ace or **F**orehead (from wasting of muscles of facial expression)
G	**G**onadal atrophy (small pituitary fossa)
H	**H**eart (cardiomyopathy/conduction defects)
I	**I**mmunology (low serum Ig) and **I**ntellectual deterioration

SWOT BOX

Myotonia (droopy eyes) is the inability of muscles to relax normally after contraction. It may be unilateral. In advanced disease it is less obvious because of muscle wasting. The resulting weakness is the main eventual cause of disability.

Myotonic dystrophy often manifests in adolescence or childhood and progresses thereafter. There is also an autosomal dominant congenital form (myotonia congenita) which can manifest itself *in utero*. To check for this, ask the patient to grip your fingers or shake your hand firmly, then let go as fast as possible. The delay in relaxation worsens in the cold and on excitation.

Parkinson's disease

TRAP is a neat way to remember the clinical features of Parkinson's.

TRAP

T	**T**remor at rest (4–7 Hz)
R	**R**igidity
A	**A**kinesia
P	**P**osture (simian) and gait (shuffling)

Peripheral neuropathy

The five main causes conveniently start with the first five letters of the alphabet.[15]

A-B-C-D-E

A	**A**lcohol
B	**B**12
C	**C**hronic renal failure and **C**arcinoma
D	**D**iabetes and **D**rugs
E	**E**very vasculitis

15 From Dr Robert Clarke (2004–2007) *Medicine for Finals*. Dr Clarke's Revision Courses in Association with the BMA.

Reflexes

This is a popular and simple aide-memoir to remember which nerves relate to which reflexes.[16]

AK-BeST

A	**A**nkle (S1)
K	**K**nee (L2, L3, L4)
BeST	**B**iceps, **S**upinator (C5, C6) and **T**riceps (C7)

SWOT BOX

All the muscles on the dorsal aspect of the upper limb are innervated by C7 – in other words, the triceps, wrist and finger extensors.

Restless legs syndrome

Considered to be a neurological sensorimotor disorder, this can be diagnosed using the URGE criteria.[17]

URGE

U	**U**rge – Is there an urge to move the legs?
R	**R**esting – Does resting bring it on?
G	**G**etting up – Does getting up and moving about help?
E	**E**venings – Are evenings worse?

JOT BOX

16 Faisal Raza, University of East Anglia.
17 Allen RP, Picchietti D, Hening WA, Trenkwalder C, Walters AS, Montplaisir J (2003) Restless legs syndrome: diagnostic criteria, special considerations, and epidemiology. *Sleep Medicine* 4:101–19.

7.9 RENAL MEDICINE AND UROLOGY

Cystinuria

A hereditary condition. Four dibasic amino acids are not reabsorbed by the proximal convoluted tubule (i.e. cystine, ornithine, arginine and lysine). Use COAL to remind you:

COAL

C	**C**ystine
O	**O**rnithine
A	**A**rginine
L	**L**ysine

SWOT BOX

The main consequence is that cystine stones are formed in the renal tract (cystine is the least soluble so it forms the stones). Note that cystine stones are seen on X-ray (but are less radiopaque than calcium stones).

DMSA and DTPA

Two important radiological investigations of renal integrity are the DMSA and DTPA scans:

- [^{99m}Tc]DMSA is bound to proximal convoluted tubules in the cortex but gives little indication of the physiological function (e.g. urine production).
- [^{99m}Tc]DTPA is given intravenously; a renogram curve shows vascular, secretory and excretory phases.

Highly technical so far, but this helps:

DTPA	**D**oes **T**he **P**hysiology
DMSA	**D**oesn't **M**ove

Phimosis or balanitis (or both)?

Phimosis is where the prepuce (foreskin) cannot be fully retracted so resembles a muzzle; the Greek *phimos* means 'muzzle'.

PHoreskin **m**uzzle = **PH**im**o**sis

Balanitis is inflammation of the glans. [Latin *glans* means 'acorn'.]

When the prepuce and glans are both affected, it is termed **balanoposthitis**.

Prostatic hypertrophy

Between a quarter and half of all men in their forties and fifties have benign prostate hypertrophy.[18]

[Think of 1/**4** to **50**% in age **40–50**]

60% of men in their **sixties**

70% of men in their **seventies**

80% of men in their **eighties**

Scrotal mass – causes

Remember the possible causes of a single scrotal mass using this mnemonic.

GHOST

G	**G**umma (nodile in tertiary stage syphilis)
H	**H**aematocele
O	**O**rchitis
s	**s**mall testes with large epidymis found in epidiymitis
T	**T**umour and **T**orsion

Testicular cancer

Younger men (age range 25–55 years) get **teratomas**. In older men **seminomas** are more common.

Troops and Sergeants[19]

Troops and	**T**eratomas
Sergeants	**S**eminomas

---

18 Data from Forte, Vincent, 'Ten Tips of Treating Enlarged Prostate', *Doctor newspaper*, June 2000.
19 Contributed by Nicola Carter, King's College London.

Urethral stricture - causes

Congenital (e.g. pinhole meatus)
Urethral valves
Neoplastic
Trauma (e.g. surgery, injury, foreign body) *and*
Inflammation (gonorrhoea, meatal ulceration)

You can use the anagram TUNIC, or a suitable equivalent as you wish.

JOT BOX

PAEDIATRICS

Apgar score

Here's a mnemonic used in daily clinical practice all over the world – a great one to show those who tell you they've never used mnemonics!

APGAR stands for **A**ppearance (colour of trunk), **P**ulse, **G**asp (respiratory effort), **A**ctivity (muscle tone), and **R**esponse to stimulation (e.g. irritating the sole).

APGAR SCORE	0	1	2
Appearance	Blue (all over)	Blue limbs	Pink
Pulse	0	< 100	> 100
Gasp	Absent	Irregular	Regular/ crying
Activity	Flaccid	Diminished; limb flexion	Active movement
Response to stimulation	None	Poor (e.g. grimace)	Good (e.g. crying)

JOT BOX

SWOT BOX

Virginia Apgar (1909–1974) was an American anaesthetist whose proposal for this scoring system was published in 1953. In 1963 the acronym APGAR was devised and coauthored with Dr J. Butterfield in the *Journal of the American Medical Association* and is one of the most utilized mnemonics in medicine.

The score is usually taken at 1 minute and at 5 minutes after delivery. A score of < 4 in the first minute indicates that intubation should be considered (especially if the score is falling). Babies with this score have a 17% mortality rate (48% if they are low birth weight); with a score of < 4 at 5 minutes, there is 44% mortality.

Blood pressure

A quick formula for normal BP *in kids* is:

$$\frac{90 + \text{age (in years)}}{55 + \text{age (in years)}}$$

Body weight

The approximate weight of a child over 1 year is given by:

$$(\text{age in years} + 4) \times 2$$

For infants up to 1 year:

Weight (kg)	Age (months)
6	3
8	6
9	9
10	12

Breastfeeding

Look at all these advantages of BREASTMILK!

BREASTMILK

B	**B**onding
R	**R**educed solute
E	**E**czema
A	**A**llergy protection
S	**S**terilization not required
T	**T**aurine
M	**M**acrophages
I	**I**mmunoglobulin A; higher **I**Q
L	**L**actoperoxidase, **L**ysosymes, **L**actoferrrin and **L**ong-chain fatty acids
K	**C**ot death (lower incidence)

Remember, too, that:

Cows' milk **C**ontains **C**asein – **C**urd protein

And that:

Human milk **H**as more w**H**ey

SWOT BOX

A milk formula will resemble human milk more closely if it has a high **whey** to **curd** ratio. Higher-curd formulas are marketed 'for hungrier babies'.

NOTE: 1 oz equals 30 ml.

Breastfed babies are protected from **allergies** and are less likely to be intolerant to cow's-milk protein. Studies show that they have a lower incidence of **eczema** and a higher **IQ** due to long-chain fatty acids in the breastmilk. **Long-chain fatty acids** are added to some formulas. Breastmilk also contains **macrophages** that kill bacteria, **lysosymes**, **lactoferrrin** which promotes **lactobacilli** and inhibits *Escherichia coli*, and **taurine**, which aids development. It also has reduced levels of **solutes** such as sodium, phosphate and proteins compared with formula milk.

Breathing (respiratory) rates

Here they are, by age:

Age	Approx. respirations/min
1 month	60
1 year	30
10 years	15

NOTE: See also the Tachycardia (pulse rate) quick rule on p. 125.

Child protection awareness: SNIPE

Five types of child abuse all health professionals need to be mindful of:

1. **S**exual abuse: Sexual activities of any sort performed upon a child by an adult (or young person able to understand what s/he is doing)

2. **N**eglect: Failure to provide for the child's basic needs

3. **I**nduced or fabricated illness

4. **P**hysical abuse or non-accidental injury (NAI)

5. **E**motional abuse: Impairing a child's emotional development or sense of self-worth (e.g. constant criticism, threats, rejection, or withholding love, support or guidance). Emotional abuse is difficult to prove but often coexists with other forms of abuse

Chromosome disorders

Three **trisomies** and their affected chromosomes:

PED

P	**P**atau's (+ 13)
E	**E**dward's (+ 18)
D	**D**own's (+ 21)

Four **chromosome deletions** to remember:

Wolf Pray, Angel Cry

Wolf	**Wolf**–Hirschhorn syndrome (4p-)
Pray	**Pra**der–Willi (chromosome 15)
Angel	**Ang**leman's (chromosome 15)
Cry	**C**ri du chat (5p-)

Conjunctivitis, neonatal

The rule of 5s 'GCS'

Age 0–5 days	exclude *Neisseria gonorrhoeae*
Age 5 days–5 weeks	exclude *Chlamydia*
Age 5 weeks–5 years	consider *Streptococcus* or *Haemophilus influenzae* type 3

N. gonorrhoeae can lead to corneal ulcers, perforation and permanent scarring, and blindness can quickly result from conjunctival infections, hence the urgent need to consider this and take eye swabs if necessary.

Cytomegalovirus

Three important facts about CMV:[1]

The three 3s of CMV

3% is the rate of primary infection (this is the commonest primary infection in pregnancy)

30% is the risk of transmission to the fetus (half are due to reactivation of the virus)

3 per 1000 births is the UK incidence

SWOT BOX

95% of affected infants with **cytomegalovirus infection** are asymptomatic, although 10% of these may become deaf in later life. There is a 30% mortality rate for those with severe congenital disease.

Complications include low birth weight, neurological sequelae, abortion, anaemia, hydrops, pneumonitis and purpura. **Investigations** include CMV on throat swab, urine, infant serum IgM. Transfusion services provide CMV-screened blood for neonates.

1 Figures from Gilbertson NJ, Walker S (1993) *Notes for the DCH*, 1st edn. Edinburgh: Churchill Livingstone.

Dehydration

Signs of severe dehydration (i.e. dehydration of 10% or more by weight in children) you need to know are low urine output, mental irritation or lethargy, and pulse either tachycardic or thread with bradycardia. There are dry mucous membranes with sunken eyes (and fontanelles in infants), prolonged capillary refill (> 3 seconds, NICE guidelines) and reduced skin turgor. It may help to remember:

10 MUPPETS

Mental signs	Irritable/shock
Urine	Output zero or negligible
Pulse	Tachycardic (think of pounding) or bradycardic/thread (think of pathetic)
Parched	Very dry mucous membranes
Eyes	Sunken
Time cap refill	> 3 seconds
Skin turgor	> 2 seconds

Developmental dysplasia of the hip

Developmental dysplasia of the hip (DDH) is associated with these risk factors:

The 7 Fs of DDH

Fetal factors (such as multiple pregnancies)

Floppy (hypotonia)

Feet first (more common in breech presentation)

First born

Female

Family history

Freezing (said to be more common in winter-born babies)

While the gold-standard screening test for dysplastic or dislocated hips in infants is the ultrasound, in UK practice most babies are not screened this way and we still rely on visual checks of symmetry of creases and Barlow's and Ortolani's tests. These tests can only be done up to about 3 months of age (too much muscle tone in limbs beyond this age makes the tests very painful).

Barlow's test is for a *dislocata**B**le* hip. The hip is flexed to 90° and adducted. Then the femoral head is pushed posteriorly, while internally rotating. A dislocatable hip will 'clunk' as it slips over the rim of the acetabulum.

Ortolani's test is for a hip that is *already dislocated*. This can be done next. The hips and knees are flexed with your middle finger over the greater trochanter and your thumb along the medial femur. Pull the hip gently forwards while abducting.

To summarize:

> **B**arlow's is **B**ackwards
> **O**rtolani's is **O**utwards

Fallot's tetralogy

Fallot's tetraology is **R**ight ventricular hypertrophy, **A**SD and **P**ulmonary stenosis – **RAP**. Then there's this:

Fella's Blue – Pull His *Vesd* Right Over

Fella's	**Fallot**'s
Blue	Cyanotic
Pull his	**Pul**monary stenosis
VeSD	**VSD** (ventricular septal defect)
Right	**Right** ventricular hypertrophy
Over	**Over**-riding aorta

SWOT BOX

Etienne-Louis Arthur Fallot (1850–1911) was Professor of Hygiene and Legal Medicine at Marseilles. However, **Fallot's tetralogy** was first described by the Danish anatomist, geologist, Catholic priest and physician Niels Stensen (1638–1686) to an Italian court. He also named the female gonad as the *ovary* (which was previously thought of as a female testis) and postulated that it was analogous to the egg-laying organ of birds.

Febrile convulsions

The Febrile 5s are useful here.

Febrile 5s

> **5** months to **5** years is approx. age range affected
> **5**% of children affected
> **5**0% recurrence rate

Gum hypertrophy

RAPID REVISION

You may remember the causes of gum hypertrophy from 'Look! Funny Crowns'. They are leukaemia, phenytoin and Crohn's or ciclosporin.

Innocent murmur

You should know the 'S' signs of an innocent murmur:

The 6 S signs

Symptom free

Systolic

Split-second sound

Sternal edge (left) side

Small part of pulmonary area only

Signs are otherwise normal

Kawasaki disease

This is also known as mucocutaneous lymph node syndrome. The CRESTS signs apply here:

CRESTS

C	**C**ervical lymphadenopathy; **C**-reactive protein raised
R	**R**ash (widespread, polymorphic)
E	**E**yes (bilateral, non-exudative conjunctivitis)
S	**S**trawberry tongue; red lips
T	**T**emperature raised (persists over 5 days, unresponsive to antibiotics and antipyretics)
S	**S**ausage-like fingers/toes from oedema **S**kin on palms/soles peeling

Mumps – still MOPE-ing??

SWOT BOX

Mumps is caused by an airborne **paramyxovirus** (and is also spread by direct contact via body fluids). Uncommon in adults, it is often subclinical in children. Salivary gland inflammation is often the principal manifestation (e.g. parotitis, either uni- or bilateral).

Complications include epididymo-orchitis, oophoritis, meningoencephalitis and pancreatitis. Mumps meningitis is usually benign (vomiting, neck rigidity, lethargy, headache, photophobia, convulsions, abdominal pain and fever).

Investigations include cerebrospinal fluid (CSF), positive throat swab, stool culture and rising titre on serum antibody.

NOTE: The MOPE mnemonic referred to was explained on p. 57. It stands for meningism, orchitis/oophoritis, parotitis/pancreatitis/paramyxovirus and encephalitis.

Nappy rash

Some of the causes are given here.

PEE-SAC

P	**P**soriasis
E	**E**czema
E	**E**xcoriation (e.g. due to diarrhoea, acid stools, disaccharide intolerance, etc.)
S	**S**eborrhoeic dermatitis
A	**A**mmoniacal dermatitis
C	**C**andidiasis

Recessive genetic disorders

Rhyme about some autosomal recessive conditions:

A sick taxi driver named **Fred**
A **Thali** he'd had before bed
Dr **Hoffman** was called
But his **girdle** was mauled
So **incysted** I **PicK U** instead!

And this is what it all means:

Fred	**Fried**reich's ataxia (see pp. 107–8)
Thali	**Thal**assemia
Hoffman	Werdnig–**Hoffman**
Girdle	Limb **girdle** dystrophy
In**cyst**ed	**Cyst**ic fibrosis
Pic**KU**	**PKU** (phenylketonuria)

Here are some **X-linked recessive disorders**:

Bright Rats with VD Are Incontinent

Bright	Al**bright** syndrome
Rats	**Rett** syndrome
VD a**Re**	**V**itamin **D**-**R**esistant rickets
Incontinent	**Incontinent**ia pigmenti

Tachycardia (pulse rate) definition[2]

Here is the quick ×10 pattern:

× 10

Children > **12** months	Normal max. HR = **120**
Children > **10** years	Normal max. HR = **100** (i.e. same as adults)

TORCH'S infections

These are important non-bacterial infections that can affect the fetus:

TORCH'S

T	**T**oxoplasmosis (see below)
O	**O**ther STDs (e.g. syphilis)
R	**R**ubella (an RNA virus)
C	**C**ytomegalovirus (see p. 142)
H	**H**erpes (e.g. chickenpox)
S	**S**lapped cheek (parvovirus B19)

---

2 See http://www.livestrong.com/article/92911-normal-pediatric-pulse-rate/#ixzz15IbJbvuV (Accessed: 24 February 2016)

Toxoplasmosis

The 'tOXO' tetrad is shown here.

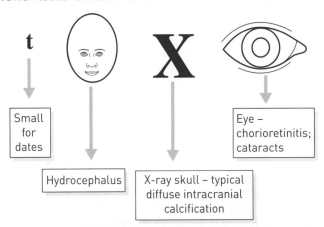

Small for dates

Hydrocephalus

X-ray skull – typical diffuse intracranial calcification

Eye – chorioretinitis; cataracts

SWOT BOX

The protozoan ***Toxoplasma gondii*** has its sexual cycle in the cat. It enters the human food chain by ingestion of oocytes (obtained via raw meat from other animals). Around 75% of the UK population are susceptible to this, but the vertical transmission rate is only 1 in 100 and only 10% of affected fetuses are damaged. Infected patients may be totally asymptomatic or may develop a non-specific illness with fatigue and flu-like symptoms.

Twelve cases are reported annually to the CDSU (Communicable Diseases Surveillance Unit). Pregnant women found to have seroconverted may be treated with 3-weekly courses of spiramycin to reduce risk to the fetus. Infected neonates may be treated with spiramycin alternating with pyrimethamine + sulfadiazine.

SURGICAL SPECIALTIES

This chapter covers general surgery and surgery within the disciplines of orthopaedics, ENT and ophthalmology.

PRE-QUIZ

1 Can you describe the branches of the renal artery?
2 What should you ask in the history of a person with jaundice?
3 Who traditionally are said to get gallstones?
4 Do you remember which eye muscles are innervated by the IIIrd cranial nerve?
5 What are the signs of an arterial thrombus?
6 Can you name the ocular sign of syphilis?
7 What features on a mole imply a high suspicion of malignancy?
8 Which non-absorbable sutures can you name?

JOT BOX

9.1 GENERAL SURGERY

A surgical sieve

VITAMIN C DIP is a sieve for aetiologies of various pathologies. It's completely daft but it works something like this:

VITAMIN C DIP

V	**V**ascular
I	**I**nfective
T	**T**rauma
A	**A**llergy/immunological
M	**M**etabolic/endocrine
I	**I**atrogenic
N	**N**eoplastic
C	**C**ongenital
D	**D**egenerative
I	**I**diopathic
P	**P**sychogenic

Here are two more old favourites:

In A Surgeon's Gown, Physicians Might Make Some Progress

In	**In**cidence
A	**A**ge
Surgeon's	**S**ex
Gown	**G**eography
Physicians	**P**redisposing factors
Might	**M**acroscopic
Make	**M**icroscopic
Some	**S**urgery
Progress	**Prog**nosis

In A Surgeon's Gown, A Physician Can Cause Inevitable Damage To Patients

In	**I**ncidence
A	**A**ge
Surgeon's	**S**ex
Gown	**G**eography
A	**A**etiology
Physician	**P**athology
Can	**C**linical presentation
Cause	**C**omplications
Inevitable	**I**nvestigations
Damage	**D**ifferential diagnosis
To	**T**reatment
Patients	**P**rognosis

Abdominal distension – causes

The 6 Fs
A **F**latulent **F**at **F**etus **F**loats in **F**luid **F**aeces

Arterial thrombus

The P signs
Pale/pallor
Painful
Pulseless
Paralysed
Paraesthesia
Perishing with cold!

Battle's sign

This is bruising behind the ear from a posterior fossa fracture. It is a sign of major trauma. W.H. Battle (1855–1936) was a surgeon at St Thomas's. Use simple pattern recognition here:

Imagine being hit on the back of the head in a battle

Breast cancer

D's nipple changes[1]

Deviation

Depression

Destruction

Displacement

Deviation

Discharge

Duplication

Burns

The rule of 9s[2]

Back of trunk	**9**% × 2
Front of trunk	**9**% × 2
Each arm	**9**%
Each leg	**9**%
Head and neck	**9**%
Perineum	1%
Hand	1%

NOTE: Do not include simple erythema in the estimate.

Central abdominal pain

If it's **acute**, here are some possible causes:

Your Terrible Ties Make Gas in Uranus

Your	**Y**ersinia
Terrible	**T**uberculosis
Ties	**T**yphoid
Make	**M**eckel's
Gas	**G**astroenteritis
IN	**IN**flammatory bowel disease (IBD)
URanus	**UR**inary tract infection

1 Modified from Browse N, Black J, Burnand KG, Thomas WEG (2005) *Browse's Introduction to Symptoms and Signs of Surgical Disease*, 4th edn. London: Arnold.
2 From Collier JAB, Longmore M, Brinsden M (1999) *Oxford Handbook of Clinical Specialties*, 5th edn. Oxford: Oxford University Press.

And if it's **chronic**, the causes may include:

Sticking Radios in Cranes Can End the Burglaries

Sticking	Adhesions
Radios	**Rad**iation
In	**I**schaemia of bowel
Cranes	**Cr**ohn's
Can	**Can**cer
End	**End**ometriosis
The **B**urglaries	**TB**

Clover leaf haemorrhoids

These are analogous to a **clover leaf** at positions 3 o'clock, 7 o'clock and 11 o'clock. External haemorrhoids are varicosities of the inferior rectal vein tributaries.

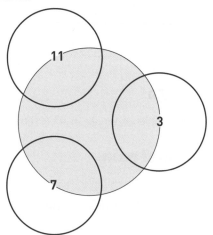

Dukes cancer staging

Dukes staging for colon cancer (modified) goes like this:

DUKES **A**	**A**-OK (best prognosis) – in bowel wall only
DUKES **B**	**B**reached **B**owel wall
DUKES **C**	**C**olonic regional nodes
DUKES **D**	**D**istant metastases

Ectropion

The eyelid goes out – think of:

Exit = **Ec**-xit

Entropion

The eyelid folds inward – remember:

IN-tropion

Gallstones

Another anonymous aide-memoire for the risk factors for gallstones.

The 5 Fs
Fair
Fat
Female
Forty
Fertile

Grey Turner's sign

This bruising of the flank(s) is a sign of retroperitoneal haemorrhage. Imagine you need to TURN them over to see it... and it is coloured GREY-ish blue.

Intestinal obstruction

Remember the symptoms like this.

Vomit PAD

Vomit	**Vomit**ing
P	**P**ain
A	**A**bsolute constipation
D	**D**istended

Jaundice

When taking a history from somebody with jaundice, you may find the mnemonic CATHODES helpful.

CATHODES

C	**C**ontacts
A	**A**naemia
T	**T**ravel
H	**H**ad it before
O	**O**perations
D	**D**rugs (including recreational intravenous use)
E	**E**xtra-hepatic causes (e.g. gallstones, sickle cell)
S	**S**exual preference

Management of cases

If you're ever in an OSCE or viva and you get stuck on a question of how to manage a case, a useful tip is TIE (backwards!):

E	**E**xplanation to the patient
I	**I**nvestigation
T	**T**reatment

While there is tea, there is hope
Sir Arthur Pinero (1855–1934)

Meckel's diverticulum

This is part of the vitello-intestinal duct which completely disappears in 98% of the population. It causes complications such as perforation, and haemorrhage from peptic ulceration, obstruction (as it contains cells similar to those from stomach or pancreas).

A Meckel's diverticulum follows this rule of 2s.

Rule of 2s

2% of the population affected
2 to 1 male to female ratio
2 inches long
2 feet from the iliocaecal valve (on the antimesenteric border of the small intestine)

SWOT BOX

J.F. Meckel the Younger (1781–1833) studied medicine in Vienna and discovered the first branchial cartilage. His grandfather first described the sphenopalatine ganglion, and his father was a Professor of Anatomy and Surgery.

Melanoma

ABCD-BITCHES helps us here. How?

A-B-C-D-BITCHES

A	**A**symmetry (irregular)
B	**B**order (notched, indistinct or ulcerated)
C	**C**olour (increasingly variegated, especially black/grey)
D	**D**epth (of invasion)
B	**B**leeding
I	**I**tching (persistent)
T	**T**ethering
C	**C**olour
H	**H**alo
E	**E**czema-like features
S	**S**ize (rapidly increasing) and **S**atellites (presence of)

Pain characteristics

Bear in mind LOST WARD as you ask about the characteristics of pain.

LOST WARD

L	**L**ocation
O	**O**nset/duration
S	**S**everity
T	**T**ransmission/radiation
W	**W**hat...
A	**A**ggravates or...
R	**R**elieves
D	**D**uration/previous diagnoses

Alternatively, try the SOCRATES approach:

SOCRATES

S	**S**ite
O	**O**nset/duration
C	**C**haracter
R	**T**ransmission/radiation
A	**A**ggravates or relieves?
T	**T**iming
E	**E**arlier diagnosis
S	**S**everity

Raynaud's phenomenon

Raynaud's disease is most common in young women (60–90% of reported cases) and is idiopathic, hence:

Raynaud's **D**isease we **D**on't know

Phenomenon has a **P**athological cause

Some of the causes are listed here, made more memorable by this naughty mnemonic.

My Servant's Vibrator's So Cold, Ergo Dame's Thighs Are Nervous

My	**M**alnutrition
Servant's	**Cer**vical rib
Vibrator's	**Vibrat**ing tools
So	**S**ubclavian aneurysm and **S**tenosis (cause emboli)
Cold	**Cold** exposure and **Col**lagen diseases
Ergo	**Ergo**t
Da**M**e's	**D**iabetes **M**ellitus
Thighs	**Thy**roid deficiency
Are	**A**therosclerosis/Buerger's disease
Nervous	**Neur**ological causes (e.g. spinal cord disease)

NOTE: Also **WBC** gives **W**hite, **B**lue and **C**rimson, the order of the sequential colour changes of the hand seen in Raynaud's phenomenon.

SWOT BOX

Raynaud's phenomenon is secondary to other conditions, such as connective tissue disorders (scleroderma, rheumatoid arthritis, systemic lupus erythematosus), obstructive arterial diseases (e.g. thoracic outlet syndrome), neurogenic lesions, drug intoxications (ergot, methysergide), dysproteinemias and myxoedema.

Sprain treatment

A very common mnemonic in clinical practice used by many health professionals.

RICE

R	**R**est
I	**I**ce (cold pack, e.g. frozen peas, or gel pack)
C	**C**ompression (tubular crepe bandage)
E	**E**levation (keep affected limb elevated)

If using ice, crush it, wrap it up in layers of towelling and apply for 10–15 minutes, but not directly to the skin. If using peas, do not eat them! Mark the bag with a big 'X' to avoid possible food poisoning.

Sutures

Here are some common types and brand names of **non-absorbable** sutures:

SLEEP

S	**S**ilk
L	**L**inen
E	**E**thilon™
E	**E**thibond
P	**P**rolene™

And some **absorbable** ones:

VCD

V	**V**icryl™ (70 days)
C	**C**atgut
D	**D**exon™

9.2 ORTHOPAEDICS

Charcot's joints

Causes of Charcot's joints to remember.

Charred lepers could syringe deaf tabby

Charred	**Char**cot's
Lepers	**Lep**rosy
Could	**C**auda equine lesion
Syringe	**Syring**omyelia (cyst in spinal cord)
Deaf	**D**iabetes
Tabby	**Tab**es dorsalis (degenerative condition of neurons)

SWOT BOX

J.M. Charcot (1825–1893) was a famous French neurologist who introduced the study of geriatrics. He also studied hypnosis and art.

Developmental dysplasia of the hip

Developmental dysplasia of the hip (DDH) is associated with the 7Fs as described on p. 120, where you will find much more on the subject. Previously this was described as congenital dislocation of the hip.

The 7 Fs of DDH

Fetal factors (such as multiple pregnancies)

Floppy (hypotonia)

Feet first (more common in breech presentation)

First born

Female

Family history

Freezing (said to be more common in winter-born babies)

Hammer or mallet toe

Hammer is a *proximal* flexion deformity, but mallet is a *distal* deformity.

Hammer (proximal) then **M**allet (distal) in alphabetical order!

Kyphosis or scoliosis?

Kyphosis is anterior curvature of the spine and *scoliosis* is lateral curvature of the spine. This picture will help you remember.

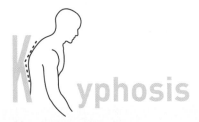

Kyphosis: *anterior curvature of the spine*

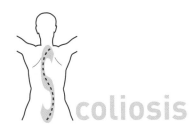

Scoliosis: *lateral curvature of the spine*

Causes of **kyphosis** are given by:

Uncle Spikes Tabby Met Oscar's Kangaroo

Uncle	**Ankyl**osing
Spikes	**Sp**ondylitis
TaBby	**TB**
Met	**Met**astatic carcinoma
Oscar's	**Os**teoporosis
Kang**a**roo	**Cong**enital

Valgum and varum

Genu *valgum* is *knock* knees and genu *varum* is *bow* knees. Can you remember that?

Valgum   Imagine GUM has GLUED the knee together

Varum   When they are bowed, the knees are *far from* each other so there is VAST ROOM (rhymes with *varum*) between the knees

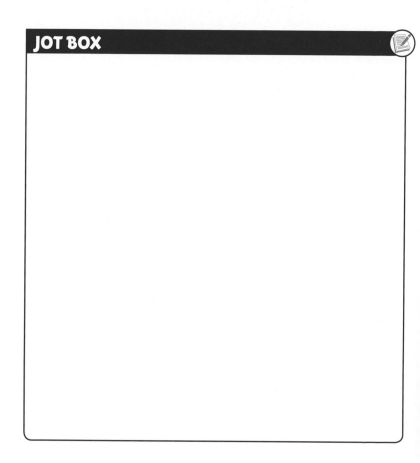

JOT BOX

9.3 EAR, NOSE AND THROAT

Cholesteatomas

It's easy to remember that cholesteatomas often lead to *attic* perforations:

Coal in the attic

SWOT BOX

This is a mass of keratinizing stratified squamous epithelium from the middle ear or mastoid cavity which can enlarge and damage or erode local tissue. It may be due to negative middle-ear pressure which then retracts the tympanic membrane – usually in the **attic** region.

Deafness

When testing for **nerve deafness**, remember:

Norm's Nerve PoWeR!

Norm's	**Norm**al ear in...
Nerve	**Nerve** deafness
PoWeR	**P**ositive **W**eber's and **R**inne's

When testing for **conductive deafness**, remember:

CD-WP

C	**C**onductive
D	**D**eafness is...
W	**W**eber's
P	**P**ositive

Rinne's and Weber's tests

In **Rinne's test** a tuning fork is applied to the mastoid, then it is placed near the ear, without any contact (held in the air). Rinne's test is a test of air conduction vs mastoid bone conduction (on the same side). A 'positive' Rinne's means the air conduction is louder than bone conduction. In Rinne's, Rs are +ve.

If Air Near Ear Is Louder, It Is Normal

ai**R**	**R**
nea**R**	**R**
ea**R**	**R**
loude**R**	**R**
no**R**mal	**R**

In **Weber's test** the tuning fork is placed once on the midline of the head (e.g. top of the head or forehead). The letter '**W**' has a *midline*. You will now know (permanently) that Weber's is the test which involves touching the tuning fork on the *middle* of the head! So, for Weber's test, remember:

W for middle

Weber's   **W** *midline* means *middle*

NOTE: In these tests, 'positive' usually means 'louder'.

JOT BOX

9.4 OPHTHALMOLOGY

Fundoscopy

Where should you look on fundoscopy?

DM-FT

DM	**D**isc is **M**edial
FT	**F**ovea is **T**emporal

Optic nerve (cranial II)

If asked to examine the function of the optic nerve, one possible scheme is AFRO.[3]

AFRO

A	**A**cuity
F	**F**ields
R	**R**eflexes (light/accommodation)
O	**O**ptic disc

NOTE: Do the optic discs *last* of all – using the bright light constricts the pupil. PERLA is an acronym for Pupils Equal and Reactive to Light and Accommodation.

Having examined the optic disc (or 'papilla'), you may see it is choking in fluid (choked disc = papilloedema). You will know this from the features CCCP.

Papilloedema

The main features of the choked disc are given by CCCP.

CCCP

C	**C**olour change...
C	**C**ontour and...
C	**C**upping imply...
P	**P**apilloedema

3 With acknowledgement to Dr Lisa Culliford of St George's Hospital Medical School.

OBSTETRICS AND GYNAECOLOGY

Antepartum haemorrhage

The causes of APH can be remembered using the acronym APH!

APH

A	**A**bruption
P	**P**lacenta praevia (or vasa praevia)
H	**H**ardly known (40% are idiopathic)

Cytomegalovirus

Remember the three 3s CMV-related facts.[1] To recap:

The three 3s of CMV

3% is the rate of primary infection

30% risk of transmission to the fetus

3 per 1000 births is the UK incidence

You'll find more information on CMV in Chapter 8, Paediatrics.

JOT BOX

---

1 Figures from Gilbertson NJ, Walker S (1993) *Notes for the DCH*, 1st edn. Edinburgh: Churchill Livingstone.

Forceps delivery

A few things to remember when forceps delivery is likely:

FORCEPS

F	**F**ully dilated
O	**O**cciput presentation
R	**R**uptured membranes
C	**C**atheter to empty bladder
E	**E**ngaged
P	**P**ain relief should be adequate
S	**S**pace/**S**cissors (episiotomy)

But can you remember which forceps to use for high, low and middle cavities? Try this:

WAK

W	**W**rigley's	Low
A	**A**nderson's	Mid
K	**K**ielland's (rotational)	High

NOTE: The use of Ventouse has largely superseded the high-cavity forceps.

Meig syndrome

Meig syndrome is an ovarian tumour associated with ascites and pleural effusion or hydrothorax. J.V. Meigs was a Professor of Gynaecology at Harvard. Think of a HAT for its main features.

HAT

H	**H**ydrothorax
A	**A**scites
T	**T**umour of ovary

Alternative

PAT where P is for Pleural effusion.

Pelvic dimensions

The following 11–12–13 rule helps you with the (approximate) ideal female pelvic dimensions. These are approximate anterior–posterior (AP) dimensions.

Pelvic dimensions 11–12–13

11 cm (AP) × 13 cm (transversely)

12 cm (mid-cavity of pelvis)

13 cm (AP) × 11 cm (transversely)

The pelvic inlet is wider transversely and the outlet is wider anteroposteriorly.

The variation in diameter through the pelvis is a human characteristic – an adaptation to bipedal stance – which helps one walk upright but makes the second stage of labour more difficult for the fetus whose head must rotate to negotiate the variable shape of the pelvic 'tunnel'.

Sperm counts – the norms

Here's a guide to the Norms (anonymous again, and apologies to Norm). Think of this as a sequence 2–2–4–6 in which the sperm count may be considered to have the following normal values:

2-2-4-6

20 million is the minimum count in....

2 ml of which at least...

40% are motile and at least...

60% have normal morphology

Sterilization counselling

These are the issues involved in counselling before FEMALE sterilization.

FEMALE

F	**F**ailure rate (1 in 500)
E	**E**ctopics (small relative increase in risk)
M	**M**enstrual changes (not taking 'the pill' any more)
A	**A**in't reversible
L	**L**aparoscopic procedure (may be done at Caesarean section if baby is healthy)
E	**E**nter in notes ('Informed of failure rate and knows irreversible')

NOTE: See Chapter 8, Paediatrics, for more information on events that can affect the fetus.

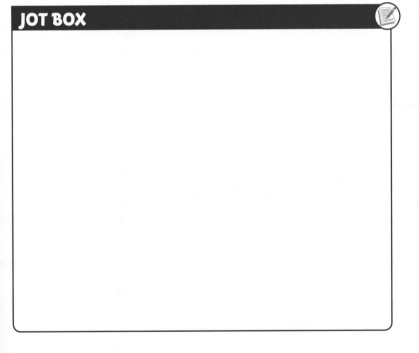

JOT BOX

PSYCHIATRY

Delusional disorders

Classification of these is simple.

Persistent Flies in Pairs Make Me Paranoid

Persistent	**Persistent** delusion disorder
Flies in	**Folie** à deux
Pairs make me	**Pa**raphrenia
Paranoid	**Paranoia**

For some special **paranoid** conditions there is:

Hypochondriac Fergi Declares Othello is Crap

Hypochondria	Monosymptomatic **hypochondria**cal psychosis (MHP)
Fergi	**Freg**oli syndrome
Declares	**De Cler**ambault syndrome
Othello is	**Othello** delusion
Crap	**Cap**gras syndrome

SWOT BOX

In **monosymptomatic hypochondriacal psychosis**, the patient is convinced there is a physical cause of complaint and 'gathers evidence' for it. **De Clerambault** syndrome is also known as *erotomania* and is the belief of one person that another person (usually unattainable) loves them intensely. People affected by **Fregoli syndrome** believe that many different people are actually the same person who changes appearance or is in disguise. The **Othello delusion** is one in which there is a belief that one's partner is unfaithful. In **Capgras syndrome**, there is a belief that a familiar person has been replaced by an exact double or an imposter.

Depression

Seven things to look out for in depression:

7 As of depression

Anhedonia
Appetite loss
Anergia
AM waking
Amenorrhoea
Asexual (decreased libido)
Affective disorder

There are eight things in this scheme of DESPAIRS:[1]

DESPAIRS

D	**D**epressed mood or disinterest
E	**E**nergy loss, TATT (tired all the time)
S	**S**leep disturbed
P	**P**essimism, hopelessness, worthlessness
A	**A**ppetite and weight change
I	**I**mpaired concentration
R	**R**etardation or agitation
S	**S**uicidal ideas or recurrent thoughts

SWOT BOX

The syndrome of depression comprises the first symptom + at least four others + significant functional impairment for > 2 weeks (preferably several weeks).

JOT BOX

1 From Kendrick T (2003) *The New Generalist* 1(2).

Mental state exam

Mad Is Pat?

M	**M**ood
A	**A**ppearance
D	**D**iet (appetite)/**D**epression
I	**I**nsight
S	**S**peech
P	**P**erceptual (sensory)
A	**A**ppearance/**A**nxiety
T	**T**houghts
?	**M**emory (concentration)

Alternative

'Pat's BMI' stands for Perceptual, Appearance, Thoughts, Speech, Behaviour, Memory/Mood, Insight.

Schizophrenia

Classification of schizophrenia is as follows:

Cats Simply Hate Parrots

Cats	**C**atatonic
Simply	**S**imple
Hate	**H**ebephrenic
Parrots	**P**aranoid

The **acute features** are:

SHADI

S	**S**tress/**S**timulation (precipitated by)
H	**H**allucinations
A	**A**ffect is incongruent
D	**D**eletions of thought
I	**I**nterference with thinking

The **chronic features** include age, disorientation, lack of volition, loosening of associations (formal thought disorder), apathy, poverty of (poor) speech and thought, blunting of affect, deteriorating social conduct (e.g. swearing in public or at staff), social withdrawal and underactivity (slowness). They are all covered in the rude poem!

NAUGHTY BIT

To a dizzy young violinist called Shadi

'Stop losing your socks, you're all apathy!'

Poor Shadi was blunt:

'Doctor, you are a ****!'

Thus withdrawing, we slowed down entirely.

The key to this verse is:

Dizzy	**Disorientated**
Young	**Age**
Violinist	**Vol**ition
Losing your socks	**Loosening** of associations
Apathy	**Apathy**
Poor	**Poverty** of speech and thought
Blunt	**Blunt**ing of affect
Withdrawing	**Withdrawal**
Slowed	**Slow**ness and underactivity

JOT BOX

RADIOLOGY

Chest X-ray

The mediastinal contours seen on chest X-ray (from top to bottom) are shown below.

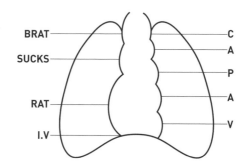

For the **right**, use:

Brat Sucks Rats IV

Brat	**B**rachiocephalic vein
Sucks	**S**VC (superior vena cava)
RATs	**R**ight **AT**rium
IV	**IV**C (inferior vena cava)

And for the **left**, use:

LAP-AV

L	**L**eft subclavian
A	**A**orta
P	**P**ulmonary artery
A	**A**trium
V	**V**entricle

Chest X-ray – congestive cardiac failure

With congestive heart failure, the chest X-ray has a bat's-wing appearance, and this is known as:

The Bat Signal

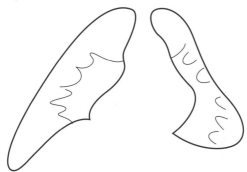

Chest X-ray – emphysema

The hyperinflated chest X-ray gives the mediastinum the typical 'strung chicken' appearance. It is:

The Strung Up Chicken of Emphysema

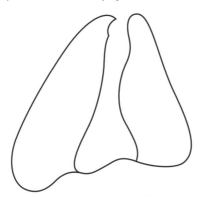

LEFT HEART FAILURE gives fluid overload in the lungs (as in XR above) – remember "**L** is for lungs".

RIGHT HEART FAILURE leads to fluid overload in other parts of the body – think "**R** for the **R**est".

Crohn's disease

You need to know the following characteristics features of CROHN'S **on X-ray**. This mnemonic was contributed anonymously.

CROHN'S

C	**C**obblestone appearance of mucosa
R	**R**ose-thorn ulcers
O	**O**bstruction of bowel
H	**H**yperplasia of mesenteric lymph nodes
N	**N**arrowing of lumen
S	**S**kip lesions (**S**arcoid foci/**S**teatorrhoea)

DEXA scans

Z score – compares bone density with someone of similar age and sex:

Z score   **Z**ame age and **Z**ex

T score – compares bone density with that of an average healthy young adult of the same sex:

T score   **T**hat young **T**hing over **T**here

Vertebral fractures

When looking for **spinal fractures on X-ray**, check for the elephant's skull – you can easily imagine two eyes and a nose. If you cannot clearly see two eyes and a nose on a particular vertebra, then it is likely to be fractured.

The Elephant's Skull

Can't see two eyes and a nose? Consider fracture

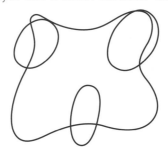

SECTION

III

STUDY TIPS AND MEMORY BITS

MISCELLANY OF MEMORY TIPS

Breaking bad news

SPIKES is a six-step protocol for delivering bad news to patients.[1]

SPIKES

S	**S**etting up
P	**P**erception
I	**I**nvitation
K	**K**nowledge
E	**E**motions
S	**S**trategy and **S**ummary

Ethics

Remember BANJO.

BANJO

B	**B**eneficence
A	**A**utonomy
N	**N**on-maleficence
J	**J**ustice
O	**O**ther

---

1 Baile WF, Buckman R et al (2000) SPIKES: A six-step protocol for delivering bad news: application to the patient with cancer. *The Oncologist* 5:302–11. See www.breakingbadnews.co.uk (Accessed 25 April 2016)

CHAPTER

14

MAKING MNEMONICS

The Big Secret of mnemonics?... Make it fun!

Mnemonics help; interest helps more. Creating mnemonics engages both brain hemispheres and keeps you focused on the material – regardless of what the actual memory aid is. Even if your mnemonic is not helpful to other people, it will have been useful to you – the act of generating a mnemonic means you are concentrating on the subject at hand.

Keep your memory aids short and sweet: (e.g. *'Mighty Ape'* for the MT–AP sequence of heart sounds is quick and easy and obvious). **Avoid long anagrams** – they only work if you know what the first letter stands for to begin with, limiting their use.

So think about a multilevel approach. For instance, look at the *first two, or even three letters*, and try to phrase a word or sentence that is relevant to the subject matter – *'Those Giant Gonads Prolong the Action'* tells you at least the first two/three letters of the anterior pituitary hormones, the phrase is in context with the topic, and it has some humour.

Seek the pattern: Consider *'Hammer Toe is Proximal to Mallet Toe'* – well, this is true, and also in **alphabetical** order. *'Two Lungs and One Heart'* uses a **numerical** pattern – there are beta-2 receptors on the lungs (2 lungs) and beta-1 receptors on the heart (1 heart).

Consider Weber's test and Rinne's test: Weber's test involves touching the tuning fork in the midline, and of course the **shape** of the first letter (W) of the word Weber has a midline – unlike the 'R' in Rinne's test. That's an easy way to distinguish them, and you'll never confuse the two again.

Listen out for any **sounds** that may give clues, as in the verse used to learn features of chronic schizophrenia in the psychiatry chapter.

Look for **visual** clues, too, such as the fact that the lower case letter 'b' looks like an upside down digit 'q' – hence, haemophilia B is due to lack of factor q.

Rude mnemonics can be very funny – but use them sparingly or you may forget who is doing what to whom and with what!

It is always a good idea to **jot your mnemonics down** (e.g. in the spaces available in this book), together with your own explanatory notes if you want, so that you can scan them rapidly the night before an exam. The act of writing them down employs **neurological recruitment** – i.e. more different neurons are involved – those of the motor cortex and visual cortex, and auditory if you say it to yourself when you do it.

And make your learning **multisensory** – **see**, **hear**, **feel**, smell and taste whenever possible, especially for the next sections where we explore the classic memory-aid concepts of *link* and *association*.

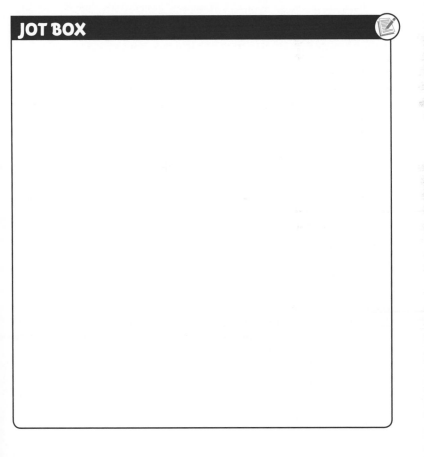

JOT BOX

LEARNING TO LINK

In the first place, association
Harry Lorayne and Jerry Lucas (*The Memory Book*)

Association is the process that links the new fact or word you don't know to something that you already know well, such as numbers, members of your family, your bedroom, etc.

We know that brain pathways are such that any word or thought can link you to a myriad of other words (see your neurology textbooks). In fact, your brain, with its hundred billion neurons, works in a non-linear fashion, like a mind map. Take, for instance, the word 'chocolate'. Instantaneously, your brain generates hundreds of associations – thoughts, ideas, words, connotations, mental images, memories and so on.

If your brain already works this way, naturally, why not use it to deliberately *associate* new facts to things you already know?

You can repeat a fact to yourself until your brain gets the message and creates a link in a random way – like, how long will that take! – or you can make it easier.

There is nothing new about association – the technique was used by the ancient Greeks to memorize key words in their long orations. They would take a mental tour around their homes, having already associated key concepts to objects they already knew. After all, you remember where your bed is and what your bathroom looks like. The phrase 'In the first place' is said to come from this practice. This is the 'loci' memory system (spatial mnemonics) and it is still used by speech-makers and memory experts (and, for example, for learning the Krebs cycle – see below).

Making associations deliberately is achieved using mental pictures. You need to exercise your imagination by producing vivid and exaggerated pictures in your mind, evoking strong imaginary emotions that are as ridiculous and out of place as possible. If you have made it this far, you already have the skills to learn a few 'advanced' memory tricks!

For instance, if a pigeon flew over your head yesterday at lunchtime, chances are you won't even remember it. But if an elephant with a striped hockey stick and yellow polka-dot boxer shorts flew over your head, you would most likely remember the image for the rest of your life! You may also remember what day it was and what you were doing at the time.

So, to learn a list, you can mentally 'link' one item to the next. Make your imaginary pictures extreme, exaggerated, ridiculous, bold, funny and outrageous. (It's okay – it's all in your head!)

Ask yourself, 'If it happened in real life, is it something I would always remember?' For example, if Martians landed in your back yard. You see, you can make it up and it will be just as memorable. Add sounds, smells and feelings to reinforce the mnemonic.

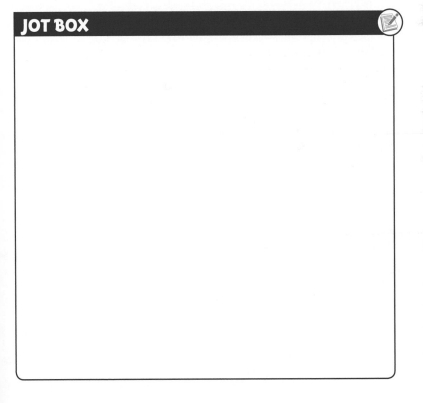

JOT BOX

THE POWER OF PEGS

... to conquer those cranial nerves

PRE-QUIZ

1 Which is the ninth cranial nerve (CN IX)?
2 Which is the seventh?
3 Which cranial nerve is the trochlear?
4 Which cranial nerve is in the abducens?
5 Which is the second?
6 Which is the twelfth?
7 List the cranial nerves **backwards** from 12ᵗʰ to 1ˢᵗ.

Having delved into the world of making associations with extreme pictures, you may now use a simple 'memory peg' to learn lists easily and reliably, in and out of sequence. But you must know how to count up to, say, 12.

First, invest the next 60 seconds memorizing this numbered list now:

1. run
2. shoe
3. tree
4. door
5. hive
6. sticks
7. heaven
8. gate
9. spine (or 'line', etc.)
10. hen
11. level crossing (or 'leaven')
12. elves (or *Twelfth Night*)

You have just learnt to use *images* to code for *number.*

Next we associate our list to the 12 pairs of cranial nerves. (You don't have to use my suggestions – your own crazy imagination works much better.)

- Cranial nerve I – **olfactory**. Imagine, say, an *oil factory* (or *oil refinery* or perhaps an *oil drilling platform*). These are 'substitute' words to help you remember the word 'olfactory'. Using substitutes facilitates visualization of vague terms. So the *oil factory* will be your analogy for the first cranial nerve (CNI). And you know that a substitute word for 1 is RUN (see list above). Let's add… movement – see, for instance, this *oil factory* growing enormous legs, like an ostrich or a dinosaur, and *running* down your street, as fast as its huge gangling, creaking bulk will allow. Close your eyes for a moment to let that picture crystallize clearly in your mind. Involve all of your senses: *smell* that crude oil (it is the first nerve after all!), *see* splodges of oil being shaken off and landing all over the place, *feel* the ground shudder with each step. We have now associated 1 with *olfactory*. Easy enough?

- Next… Cranial nerve II or 2 is the **optic** and 2 codes for SHOE. Visualize wearing *shoes* instead of *glasses* (optics), or maybe smashing a pair of *optics* by stamping on them with your favourite, newest, most expensive shoes. See that vivid image, and now exaggerate it beyond belief – make those optics shatter into millions of pieces which fly up and gather into a whirlpool of whizzing optics while your shoe continues on relentlessly…

- IIIrd CN is the **oculomotor.** Imagine your TREE (= three) with **motor**ized branches, and maybe at the end of each branch is an *eye (oculus)*. The eyes are clicking and whirring on those motorized branches, all focusing and staring at you – hundreds of motorized eyes looking straight into yours… and yet you have an unusual feeling of well-being as you realize these are your creation, entirely safe within your mind's *oculus,* with you in total control. Make the motorized branches dance and whirl as they click and spin. Got the picture? If not, make up another one!

- CNIV is the **trochlear**. We use DOOR to represent the number 4. Not just *any* door, but one that is meaningful to you – e.g. your own front door or that of somebody close to you. A substitute word for trochlear may be *truck* or *trog* (or even a pulley if you know that *trochilia* is Greek for a pulley). The possibilities are now limitless! Whatever you decide, make the image bright, bold, and noisy and exaggerated in every sense.

- The substitute word for 5 is HIVE. Nerve V is the **trigeminal**. You may, for instance, visualize an enormous hive, but instead of bees or wasps imagine of lots of precious *gems* buzzing around the hive; see them whizzing in and out and flying about your ears as they sparkle and shine. Make it so ridiculous that *if you saw it in real life, you would remember it forever.* Or you can use the word 'Gemini' for 'Trigeminal', with triplets (instead of twins) and then link those triplets to HIVE. Or whatever forms *your* associations in the most memorable way.

- Number 6 transposes to STICKS. CNVI is the **abducens.** You can use a simple picture such as *abducting* your arms with a big *stick*; make the image really vivid and multisensory.

- The number 7 = HEAVEN and the VIIth cranial nerve is the **facial** nerve. You can graphically visualize many faces, including your own, falling down from the sky (heaven). See in detail the expressions on these millions of faces as they keep falling down relentlessly – large faces, small faces... Also try imagining cloud-shaped faces floating in the sky, perhaps some are laughing, some are frowning, and some are smiling, etc.

- We now need to link the number 8 (GATE) to the **vestibulocochlear** nerve (VIII) to possible mnemonic lists, such as movies you know well... or watch as many movies as you can that you love, or videos of sporting events and finals (see p. 168). So see a gate in your mind, not just *any* gate, but a gate of importance to you, such as your own front gate, or perhaps one on a building you admire. Alternatively, you may see a *giant ear* in place of the *gate* which you have to push aside in order to get through the gate.

- Let's link 9 (SPINE) to the **glossopharyngeal** nerve. You will have the hang of it by now. One suggestion might be a giant *pharynx* in place of a spine – and it's *glossy*. Give it a good dose of pharyngitis. *Hear* it sound hoarse and make it *look* very sore and phlegmy.

- Number 10 is HEN. See an enormous hen perhaps laying an egg – make the hen look suitably *vague* for the **vagus** (or dress it up like a *magus*). Maybe a hen on the cover of *Vogue* magazine would work for you. Or whatever...

- For number 11 you could instead visualize a LEVEL CROSSING for this number. Cranial nerve XI is the **accessory** nerve. You decide which type of *accessories* to use here.

- For number 12 think of ELVEs. Imagine a dozen elves with giant *tongues* hanging out. Perhaps they are all experiencing *hypos* because they are unable to eat because of the size of their giant tongues. This should be sufficient to remind you of the **hypoglossal** nerve.

IMPORTANT: Now run through those silly images two or three more times during the next couple of minutes. So now we have:

- run – olfactory (*see* the mental picture you made)
- shoe – optic
- tree – oculomotor
- door – trochlear
- hive – trigeminal
- sticks – abducens
- heaven – facial
- gate – vestibulocochlear
- spine – glossopharyngeal
- hen – vagus
- level crossing (or leaven) – accessory
- elves – hypoglossal.

Run through this list, from the top to the bottom, in your head a couple more times, then do it **backwards**.

Now we are ready for a test!

Which is the seventh nerve? (Think of number seven; see the picture that you imagined, e.g. faces in the sky. Note how you link this picture to what represents a…facial nerve. And you know it is the seventh nerve. *How cool is that?*)

Okay, now try these:

- Which is the eleventh nerve?
- Which cranial nerve is the oculomotor?
- Which cranial nerve is in the abducens?
- Which is the first cranial nerve?

How easy was that! Oh… even if you didn't stop to review things along the way as instructed (and I'm pretty sure you didn't), you would still have got most of these correct!

Congratulations! You now know the cranial nerves in and out of order, and you also know the number assigned to them, in and out of order too! You did this with ease and loads of fun. Review them a few more times now in order to cement them into your long-term memory.

NOTE: You know the best part? After using this several times you will no longer require the actual mnemonics!

Imagination is more important than knowledge
Albert Einstein

SPATIAL MNEMONICS

Krebs cycle in your kitchen

Sometimes described as the 'loci' system of memory (Greek *locus* meaning place), spatial mnemonics were used for thousands of years as a memory aid but possibly lost popularity with the arrival of the printing press. Cicero in 516 BC documents how the poet Simonides escaped from a collapsed building where he was dining. By recalling where the many other public figures had been seated, he named all of the deceased. So this powerful method uses locations of fixed reference objects to *link–associate* what you already know (e.g. what your bedroom looks like) to what you wish to learn (e.g. the biochemical cycles).

Not too dissimilar are the oral memory traditions of many cultures whereby major events from a particular year (e.g. a flood or a storm) are linked to other happenings. Frances Yates gives a detailed account in his book *The Art of Memory* (Chicago: University of Chicago Press, 1966).

Once you learn how, with the example given below, you can apply these techniques to anything you wish.

Spatial mnemonics in 7 minutes

Link the new fact or word you need to learn (e.g. the Krebs cycle) with information that you *already remember* (e.g. your kitchen, your journey to college, members of your family, your bedroom, etc.). This process of *linking* helps us associate one bit of info with another. On pp. 43–54 you learned the actions of beta blockers by linking the facts to parts of your own body. Earlier we discussed making those extreme, exaggerated mental links and associations.

Ask yourself: If it happened in real life, is it something I would always remember?

For instance, you might conjure up a huge, smelly, red rhinoceros kissing your nose. Whatever you make up should be just as memorable.

KK's six steps to spatial mnemonics

1. **Start at a fixed point** – e.g. the DOOR or entrance.
2. **Go clockwise** around the room (or from beginning to end if it is a journey or route that you are using).
3. **Link the chunk of information you wish to learn** to the object you will always remember (whether it is your bedroom door or kitchen fridge). If you can remember where these fixed reference points are, then you can succeed at spatial mnemonics. Make your mental associations extreme, exaggerated, silly, ridiculous, dramatic and *always* over-the-top. You may also add some movement or action (remember the rhinoceros?) to the scene.
4. **Finish back at the door** – your starting point – so you know that you have completed the topic.
5. **Review** by walking around the room (this can be done *virtually,* as in the example below, but it's probably better if you can actually be in the same place). Imagine your mnemonic unfolding in front of you. Review a few times in other locations, like the bus stop and hairdressers. Make day-dreaming productive!
6. **Revise** by making notes (e.g. write it down, tabulate it, mindmap it, use rough sketches or diagrams). Closer to exam time, revise from these notes you made on the mnemonic! Teaching your friends the day before helps you to revise. You don't have to mention that you are using spatial mnemonics if you want to show off – but beware though! Your superb recall may make you less popular!

Your imagination… is worth more than you imagine
After French writer Louis Aragon

Spatial mnemonic for the Krebs cycle

Here is the tricarboxylic acid (TCA) or Krebs cycle. Try it out in your kitchen!

Oxaloacetate	(4 carbon)
Citrate	(6 carbon)
Isocitrate	(6 carbon)
Ketoglutarate	(5 carbon)
Succinyl co-A	(4 carbon)
Succinate	(4 carbon)
Fumarate	(4 carbon)
Malate	(4 carbon)

- **Start at a fixed point.** We will start at the kitchen door. Think of your chosen kitchen door. What colour and texture is it? What is it made of? Wood or glass? It may be just a doorway.

- Now link the door to the title, i.e. Krebs cycle. We can use a substitute word like 'crabs'. So imagine a huge, mighty crab guarding the kitchen entrance, snapping away at you with its mighty pincers. Notice the bright colours and contours of its shell…

- Did you notice I emphasized a *mighty* crab? This is because Krebs occurs in the mitochondrion. I just threw in an extra mnemonic for the same price! Get the picture? Good. Now make it more vivid and *turn up the volume!*

- Working our way clockwise on our mental tour around the room, the next object is the cooker. For this demonstration, we need to link **oxaloacetate** (four-carbon compound) to the cooker – how about an *ox* on the cooker? Imagine an ox is sitting on it... oxaloacetate...Wrap it in two layers of *acetate* so the two carbons – acetate – are then added. And the cooker has four hobs so emphasize that.

- Now link one of the cupboards… to **citrate**. We continue the story by opening the cupboard, from which *citrus* juice floods out, making our *eye sore* – **isocitrate**? So far so good – stay with me. We *blow* the juice off our sore eyes, hence blowing off our CO_2, which *loses us a carbon,* the next item – the *cat* eating *glue* in the microwave – **alpha-ketoglutarate**. You *dive* (= five) to save the cat and blow it out and *lose another carbon* as CO_2 – taking you to the sink.

- *Sucking coal* in the *sink*? Yep, it's **succinyl Co-A**, for sure.

- And next to that is the dishwasher – where you are sucking an 8-ball. To make it **succinate**.

- Then there is **fumarate** – the *fuming* kettle.

- Then **malate** – *mole ate* the bin.
- And after that, we are back at the beginning, in the doorway, with the *mighty crab*.

Congratulations! You have just completed your first spatial mnemonic, memorizing the Krebs cycle (*including* the numbers of carbon atoms) and you did it in somebody else's virtual kitchen! If any steps are unclear, go back and reinforce them. The technique generally works better with your own mnemonics in your own environment, where your own belongings are more familiar – think just how much more powerful this would be in a kitchen you are familiar with.

What we need to learn	Fixed reference points (examples as given above)	Your kitchen's fixed reference points (fill in as you sit in the kitchen)	Your spatial mnemonic (e.g. a mighty crab guarding the door)	Example as given above
Krebs cycle steps	Door/ entrance	Door/entrance (start here and work clockwise)		Mighty crab guarding door
Oxaloacetate	Cooker			Ox on cooker with four hobs, wrapped in acetate × 2
Citrate	Cupboards			Citrus fruits
Isocitrate	Opened the cupboards			Made your eye sore
Alpha-ketoglutarate	Microwave			Cat eating glue in microwave
Succinyl Co-A	Sink			Sucking coal in sink
Succinate	Dishwasher			Sucking an 8-ball
Fumarate	Kettle			Fuming kettle
Malate	Bin			Mole ate the bin
Back to beginning	Doorway			

REVISE AT THE MOVIES!

More links and loci

You now know that memory consists of linking what we want to know with what we already know – and as you can associate anything to anything else, it is possible to use your favourite movies, soap or sporting event to revise. People often remember their favourite movie or sporting event in remarkable detail. Why not put that to good use? Make use of movies, events and football teams that you already know by heart. The more detail you know, the more facts you can associate into your key scenes, characters, players, sportsmen and so on.

We will explore how to make use of a memory we already have to learn something we need for our exams!

I use as our example *The Wizard of Oz* (by L. Frank Baum) on the assumption that it is likely to be familiar to all or most of our readers. If you somehow have managed *not* to see this film, then go and watch it now – it is essential for your revision!

Now you already know how to link memories consciously – by associating them to something you already know, by exaggerated use of your imagination. (If you don't already know how, then go and read the last chapter, you skiver! Honestly!)

So what to learn? As an example, just for the heck of it, why not learn the peripheral somatosensory system pain and temperature pathway? As these pathways are quite awkward to learn, you may as well get it out of the way now.

Of course, you can use *any other* list or topic you wish; this book is your willing slave, after all – not the other way round! Here goes.

The peripheral somatosensory system pain and temperature pathway

- **Receptors** are in the dermis/epidermis of skin (arranged in overlapping **dermatomes).**

- Sensory neurons travel to the **dorsal root ganglion**. (A few branches will travel up or down a segment and enter the dorsal horn at a different level – this allows **overlap**.)

- The nerve synapses in the **dorsal horn** of the spinal cord.

- The second (postganglionic) neuron now **crosses over** to the contralateral side in the **ventral white matter**.

- Then it ascends in the lateral white matter.

- Some short **secondary internuncial neurons** – they connect with motor neurons to form the **reflex arc**. By the way, 'internuncial' refers to 'linking' neurons – which is exactly what you are doing now.

- Back to the collection of crossed fibres – the **lateral spinothalamic tract**.

- They travel to the **thalamus** where they synapse in the **ventral posterolateral nucleus** (VPL).

- Tertiary neurons now go to the **postcentral gyrus** (area 3, 1, 2) of the cortex – the main somatic sensory area of the brain.

I have selected a few key words here – once we have a group of key words we can begin constructing a mnemonic-based memory aid.

Back to *The Wizard of Oz*! We need the key events from the story. Briefly:

- Dorothy lives on a farm in Kansas with her dog, Toto
- House is blown away in a tornado
- House crash-lands in Oz
- Munchkins
- Glinda the Good Witch enters
- Glinda gives Dorothy a pair of ruby slippers
- Dorothy follows the Yellow Brick Road
- Meets the scarecrow who wants a brain
- Meets the tin woodman who needs oiling and a heart
- Meets the cowardly lion
- Have nice snoozy time in field of scarlet poppies (quite advanced, I thought, for a kiddie's movie, but then maybe I am showing my age!)

- Emerald City – wear emerald glasses
- Meet the Wizard…
- … who sends them off to defeat the Wicked Witch of the West
- Travel through dark enchanted forest
- Carried to the horrible witch by winged monkeys
- Dorothy melts witch with bucket of water
- Oz turns out to be fake wizard with big balloon
- Dorothy clicks heels together to get home

So now all you need to do is link *what you need to know* with *what you already know* about *The Wizard of Oz*. I have put in one or two suggestions, but now *you* have to do some of the dreamwork – it's much more fun than normal work. Once you have learned the principle, you can use it with other movies or soap operas, the FA Cup final or World Cup 1966, or whatever.

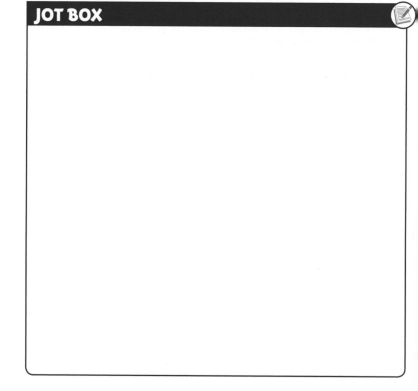

JOT BOX

What you know already	Facts you need to learn	Dreamwork (my suggestions – but make your own notes)
KANSAS, FARM	Pain and temperatures	Very hot on farm. Exaggerate the image beyond belief!
TORNADO	Start with PAIN and temperature in the dermis	Tornado blows off all of Toto's and Dorothy's dermis and epidermis
CRASH-LAND	Dorsal root ganglion	Crash on back of (dorsum) of a gang of Munchkins? Make the pictures vivid, put in sound and colour and sensations
MUNCHKINS		
GLINDA/RUBY SLIPPERS	Branches overlapping up/down a level	So many slippers that slippers are overlapping with her shoes
YELLOW BRICK ROAD	Synapse, dorsal horn	If you haven't read the previous chapter by this stage, you may be a little lost – go back now!
SCARECROW	Crossing over	Make your own images, outrageous and whacky ones
TINMAN		
LION		The rule is one mnemonic per movie!
SCARLET POPPY FIELD	Ascending in the lateral white matter	etc....
EMERALD CITY	Short neurons form the reflex arc	
WIZARD OF OZ	Lateral spinothalamic tract	
DARK FOREST	Thalamus	
WINGED MONKEYS	Synapse in VPL	
WITCH MELTING	Postcentral gyrus	
BOGUS WIZARD FLIES OFF IN BALLOON	Near the central fissure	
CLICK HEELS THREE TIMES	Area 3, 1, 2	Dorothy counts 3-1-2 as she clicks her heels, but she's a bit dizzy and gets the numbers out of order

Homework (dreamwork)!

Now that you are getting the hang of it:

- Go and watch a movie... one that you know and love really well; one in which you always remember the main scenes or characters. Being able to pause the scenes makes it even easier.

- Make a list of other memorable events you know really well like weddings, football matches, hockey finals, etc.

- Try using routes too, maybe your route to college – you may have done it hundreds of times and know it backwards (this is the loci system again).

- Try making lists of other things you know, perhaps of your flatmates, characters in your bridge club, or whatever.

- Pick a few topics in which sequences are important and dig out the *key words* – this is one of the most important stages because it makes you *summarize* and *review* as you do so. And you'll remember that summarizing and reviewing are the two most important revision skills, regardless of *how* you do them.

- Make a table like the one above, and jot down in rough your mental imagery. Or you can use a mind map.

- When revision time comes, you will only need to revise your jotted-down notes on your mnemonic and not pile through pages of text – a serious time-saver for 'night-before' revision!

Enjoy!

JOT BOX

NOOTROPICS

'Smart drugs' – and smart alternatives

Nootropics (Greek *noos* means mind and *tropos* means change) or 'cognitive enhancers' are 'a reality and people are using them', reported Susan Watts in *New Scientist* in 2011.[1] A 2013 review in the *Pharmaceutical Journal* concluded that 'popping a pill... may become the norm'.[2]

Reports suggest that 'smart drugs' may be widely used, with some students feeling obliged to take them to keep up with their peers. There is limited evidence for their effectiveness and a lack of knowledge about the long-term effects of their use. In 2015, UK Health Secretary Jeremy Hunt (Oxford alumnus) described them as 'very dangerous'.

The notes below are intended for information purposes only (most of the information is in your pharmacology texts and lectures) and the author is not condoning unlicensed use of medicinal products.

Atomoxetine

This is a noradrenalin uptake inhibitor used for ADHD treatment. It has no dopaminergic effect, hence low addiction potential. However, adverse effects include cardiac problems, aggression and psychosis. It is a prescription-only medicine (POM) and should be avoided unless prescribed on medical advice.

Caffeine

A popular trimethylxanthine, caffeine is the world's most widely used stimulant drug (ever since an Ethiopian shepherd boy discovered that coffee beans energized his flock). This CNS adenosine antagonist reduces fatigue and drowsiness and enhances alertness and coordination.[3]

---

1 Watts S (2011) The dope on mental enhancement. *New Scientist*, issue 2839, 19 November 2011.
2 *Pharmaceutical Journal*, vol. 290, 23 February 2013.
3 Personal communication.

Caffeine is legal and safe but excessive amounts should be avoided (e.g. > 200 mg per day in pregnancy or > 1000 mg per day for other adults), as they may cause diuresis, abdominal cramps, diarrhoea and anxiety. Caffeine in the late afternoon/evening can cause insomnia. This may be the effect that you want, but bear in mind what time of day your exam will be!

Tea and coffee have surprisingly similar amounts of caffeine (40–100 mg per cup) but the caffeine in tea is bound to tannins, giving a 'prolonged release' effect (up to 16 hours), while coffee tends to give you a more 'instant' hit. Green tea (from the same plant as black tea) also contains similar amounts of caffeine but the stimulant effects are counteracted by the relaxing effects of theanine.

TEA TIP 1: To reduce the amount of caffeine in tea, add hot water then discard the water, add a second infusion of hot water, then make your tea as usual. Tea expert Don Mei from the AcuMedic Foundation, London, points out that caffeine is highly water soluble and will dissolve out quickly compared with other phytochemicals, so discarding the first 30-second infusion reduces the total caffeine dose in a cup of black tea, by about 20–30%.[4]

TEA TIP 2: You can make a mug of coffee with a tea bag at the same time. This produces a strong beverage which gives you instant caffeine release followed by a longer caffeine action over several hours. A half teaspoon of wild honey improves the taste.

Donepezil

Used in the treatment of Alzheimer's disease, donepezil helps attention and memory. It is a piperidine-based non-competitive reversible inhibitor of acetylcholinesterase (ACh). It is available only on prescription (POM) and cognitive benefits appear to be limited to a small cohort of patients where symptoms are caused by ACh deficiency in the first place. It has the usual cholinergic side effects (increased secretions, diarrhoea, vomiting, etc.) and also insomnia. One study by Balsters and colleagues showed that donepezil actually impaired memory in healthy (older) subjects.[5]

Exercise

Exercise comes with a plethora of solid evidence backing the cognitive benefits as well as many pleiotropic benefits. Professor Barbara Sahakian,

---

4 Don Mei, personal communication.
5 Balsters JH, O'Connell RG, Martin MP et al (2011) Donepezil impairs memory in healthy older subjects: behavioural, EEG and simultaneous EEG/fMRI biomarkers. *PLoS One* 6(9):e24126.

a leading authority on nootropics from Cambridge University, describes exercise as being the most effective, best-documented and safest cognitive enhancer.[6]

Ginseng *(Panax ginseng)*

Panax ginseng root (and a variety of related species loosely referred to as ginseng) derived from traditional Chinese medicine has been shown to have cognitive benefits.[7] Korean ginseng is considered to be the finest. Ginseng is legal, safe and readily available.

TIP: If you decide to trial herbal medicines, they are best obtained from a supplier who can also give individual advice. (Traditionally, ginseng root is considered to be more appropriate for males than females, for whom white angelica root is a suitable equivalent. However, there seems to be insufficient evidence at the time of writing pertaining to angelica as a nootropic.)

Guarana

This is a South American herbal extract naturally high in caffeine. See **Caffeine** above.

Hayfever meds – antihistamines and decongestants

It's an unfortunate fact that many major university exams take place at the height of the hay fever season. To make matters worse, in large cities the effects are augmented by traffic pollutant particles which stick to the pollen grains (like fluff on balls of Velcro®), making them ideal delivery vehicles for sending toxins into your respiratory tract. The end result may be anything from slight sniffles to severe allergy symptoms, just when you need to be at your best. Mouth breathing secondary to rhinitis also leads to a host of additional symptoms such as pharyngitis, tonsillitis, tiredness and even sleep apnoea. So, for those affected students, it is smart to be prepared – don't lose marks to common allergies!

Recommended anti-histamines include fexofenadine and loratadine, which are considered to be 'non-drowsy' meds. If you are experiencing

---

6 Turner DC, Robbins TW, Clark L, Aron AR, Dowson J, Sahakian BJ, University of Cambridge (2003) Cognitive enhancing effects of modafinil in healthy volunteers. *Psychopharmacology (Berlin)* 165(3):260–9.

7 For example, see research from Northumbria University: Reay JL, Kennedy DO, Scholey AB (2005) Single doses of *Panax ginseng* (G115) reduce blood glucose levels and improve cognitive performance during sustained mental activity. *Journal of Psychopharmacology* 19(4):357–65.

any nasal/sinus congestion, also consider decongestants such as pseudoephedrine syrup or tablets. Take these in the morning or early afternoon (but not late because they may keep you awake).

TIP: Remember that pseudoephedrine is for short-term (up to 5 days)/ occasional use at the lowest effective dose. Pseudoephedrine and antihistamines make a sensible combination because, in theory, the drowsiness effected by antihistamines is counteracted by the alertness-raising potential of pseudoephedrine (it is banned in sports), however I can provide no evidence for this or for pseudoephedrine as a cognitive enhancer. Also long-term use raises blood pressure – and your pharmacist may wonder if you're making crystal meth in your spare time (which is neither legal nor recommended)!

Methylphenidate

Methylphenidate is a CNS stimulant that inhibits dopamine re-uptake, which accounts for most of its euphoric and addictive actions. Reports suggest that it is one of the more widely available nootropics; some students have these legitimately prescribed for treatment of their ADHD. It is based on amphetamine ('speed') and is a schedule 2 controlled drug. Nicknames include 'ritie', 'vitamin R', and 'kiddie cocaine' (because it has been used nasally to produce a similar 'high'). Adverse effects include cardiotoxicity, behavioural problems and, of course, addiction. There is no evidence to suggest that methylphenidate brings any significant benefits during exams but many anecdotal reports of problems associated with misuse.

Modafinil (Provigil®)

Modafinil promotes wakefulness and reduces fatigue and sleepiness. Its legal status is POM – legal to use/possess/buy; it is licensed only for narcolepsy in Europe. The drug's action probably involves GABA, glutamate and hypocretin. Reported uses include aviation, military and for astronauts, and students and journalists have used modafinil to stay awake, putting off sleep in order to get tasks done. Researchers at the University of Cambridge have also studied shift workers, paramedics and surgeons. Known side effects are mainly gastrointestinal, but also skin rashes, anxiety and headaches. A 2015 study in *European Neuropsychopharmacology* considered modafinil to be generally safe.[8]

---

8 Battleday RM, Brem AK (2016) Modafinil for cognitive neuroenhancement in healthy non-sleep-deprived subjects: A systematic review. *European Neuropsychopharmacology* 26(2):391.

To summarize, the evidence suggests that modafinil makes the subject more alert and energetic but that it has no significant advantages over caffeine.[9]

Omega-3

Several studies suggest that omega-3 supplements ('clever capsules') boost exam performance, possibly by optimizing myelin sheath health. Average Western diets are relatively low in omega-3. There seems to be less evidence that this helps in those who already have adequate nutritional intake of fish oil. Given the pathetic state of most student diets, and with omega-3 easily available and legal, it is worth considering as a supplement, especially for the last 3 months leading to major exams unless you already have a diet rich in oily fish, walnuts and flax seeds. The review conducted by Amanda Kirby and colleagues is a useful source of further information.[10]

Taurine

An amino sulfonic acid derived from cysteine, taurine is naturally present in meat and fish (so levels may be low in vegans), is essential for skeletal muscle and CNS function, and is present in bile. Although it is a common ingredient in energy drinks (e.g. Red Bull[11]) and body-building supplements, taurine has been shown to have an anxiolytic, calming effect which may make it useful to offset pre-exam stress.

Tea of peppermint and scent of rosemary

According to a study by Dr Mark Moss, Robert Jones and Lucy Moss of Northumbria University, **peppermint tea** (taken twenty minutes before testing) significantly improves long-term and working memory in healthy adults.

Meanwhile, Emma McCready, from the same department, and Dr Mark Moss found that the aroma of **rosemary essential oil** (via diffuser) may improve prospective memory in healthy adults.[12] This confirms what folklore has taught us for centuries.

9 Wesensten NJ, Belenky G, Kautz MA, Thorne DR, Reichardt RM, Balkin TJ (2002) Maintaining alertness and performance during sleep deprivation: modafinil versus caffeine. *Psychopharmacology (Berlin)* 159(3):238–47.
   Turner DC, Robbins TW, Clark L, Aron AR, Dowson J, Sahakian BJ, University of Cambridge (2003) Cognitive enhancing effects of modafinil in healthy volunteers. *Psychopharmacology (Berlin)* 165(3):260–9.
   The 2002 review by Wesensten et al. suggested no significant benefit over a placebo; Turner et al. (2003) found that subjects were more 'alert, attentive and energetic', but they found no significant effects on spatial memory or visual information processing.
10 Kirby A, Woodward A, Jackson, S (2009) Benefits of omega-3 supplementation for school children: review of the current evidence. *British Journal of Educational Research*. First published 24 July 2009 (iFirst). doi: 10.1080/01411920903111557
11 Seidl R, Peyrl A, Nicham R, Hauser E (2000) A taurine and caffeine-containing drink stimulates cognitive performance and well-being. *Amino Acids* 19(3–4):635–42.
12 Annual Conference of the British Psychological Society, Nottingham, April 2016.

20

MOTIVATIONAL BITS, QUIPS AND STUDY TIPS

A potpourri of thoughts, ideas, musings and wisdom, ancient and modern, together with a soupçon of solidly useful study tips to see you on your way…

Suddenly the euphoria of being at university is gone; there is an eerie silence in the air; where once there was laughter and milling throngs, all around is despair. And worst of all is the weird sensation that, even though you are surrounded by hundreds of other people, you are almost alone… Yep, it's exam season again!

Well, like I said, *almost* alone – now is the time you find out who your friends really are – and you will have discovered that this little book is up there with the best of them!

So strap yourself into that chair/couch/bed, put the kettle on and prepare to share the wisdom of some of the world's finest thinkers – and as you meld in this way remember that you, too, are among them!

> *The surest way to be late is have plenty of time*
> Leo Kennedy

Breaks and time outs

Have regular breaks! This is evidence-based, folks – you retain more and work more productively if you have sensible rest or gaps during your challenging schedule.

Say for a full day of study:

- Start off with breaks of 10–20 minutes each hour when you are fresh.
- Be flexible with your breaks – with experience, your own body will tell you what feels right.
- Then, as the hours pass by and your interest starts flagging, you may need to increase the break times in order to keep you studying efficiently.
- So, by the evening, you may have half an hour of swotting followed by a half-hour break.
- Before you start your break, run through in your mind what you have just done, for a few seconds only – so you rapidly skim through main headings and points at high speed.
- When you come back from your break, rapidly skim through the stuff you did previously, in your mind's eye, again for a few seconds. This sets you up quickly to get back into 'mode'.

This way in any 12-hour period you will get several hours' productive revision done. Working flat out without a break only gives you useful revision for the first few hours; after that you become tired, possibly lose interest, and your learning starts flagging. Twelve hours straight without a break is very inefficient compared with the same period with realistic, generous and regular breaks.

Remember to eat too!

Buddies

Hopefully, you can surround yourself with a good group of revision buddies. It helps to teach each other different parts of the syllabus (hugely time saving). You will have your own individual strategy of course.

Caffeine

Caffeine is certainly extremely useful as a mild stimulant – but beware of overdoing it as it can only give you so much of a lift before the shakes start, and diuresis (not helpful to you during exams) and, even worse, diarrhoea and wind (not helpful to the person in the chair behind you).

Sleep deprivation is also unhelpful. And remember that caffeine may stay in your system for hours, so even when you do sleep, it will reduce the overall quality of that sleep and may result in that 'Why am I tired all the time if I am having loads of caffeine?' syndrome. Be good to yourself. And set realistic goals (see below).

Common? How common *is* common?

Remember this if you're ever stuck for figures:

1 : 30	Common
1 : 300	Uncommon
1 : 3000	Rare

Environment

Learning is a process by which your brain makes certain neurological connections. Everything happening to you at the time you learn adds a few sub-branches to that particular connection in your neural network (see your neurology texts). With 100 billion neurons in your brain, the number of possible neuronal combinations is greater than the number of atoms in the universe!

And there's more – your brain is a self-evolving organ, constantly remodelling itself to adapt to all the challenges that you throw at it.

Your immediate learning environment is part of your revision also. If you are doped up on caffeine while revising, your brain remembers that too. When you need to reproduce the information in your exam with no caffeine in your bloodstream, your brain will find it that much harder to access the facts you need.

In other words, aim to match aspects of your environment – including biochemical factors – to simulate as closely as possible the exam conditions. You might even be able to revise the subject in the room where you will be taking the exam. If this is not possible, then you can use different rooms for different subjects (so that thinking of a specific room, what it looks and feels like, will act as a memory jogger). This also helps reduce confusion between different subjects.

You may have heard about students who could only pass exams while having a raised blood ethanol level, who are useless while sober! Now you know why.

So try to make sure that your blood levels of caffeine and glucose are the same as they will be during the exam. If certain music helps you to remember but you are then not allowed to wear personal stereos during the exam, beware! (If there is no other option, listen to your music on the journey to the exam centre.) Take whatever sensible and logical steps you can – then go for it!

Goal-setting

- Define your study goals/amounts/times before you start.
- Make your goals SMART.

RAPID REVISION

SMART goals are:

S   **S**pecific and **S**imple

M   **M**easurable and **M**eaningful

A   **A**ll relevant areas

R   **R**ealistic and **R**esponsible

T   **T**imed toward what you want

- Give yourself *realistic* targets – learn *smarter*. Time is limited (both for you and your swotty neighbour). If it won't help you pass, then ignore it! As Emerson said, 'Life is too short!'
- Define your *break times*. A countdown timer is useful and can be found on most digital watches, microwaves and kitchen appliances.
- *Allow for roughly 2 minutes' overview at the beginning and end of each session.*
- Decide what you will learn *now* and what you will cover *later* – when and if you have the time. This is called *prioritizing* your resources, and it is a skill that is especially important to doctors.
- Define goals for the session, the day, the term, the year – or even set lifelong targets! The use of goals and targets has permeated all walks of life, from fiscal to political, motivational and self-development for the simple reason that *goal-setting works!* Write down your goals, aims and objectives.
- However, if your dominant thoughts are about a football match, a movie or going out – good news! *It is still possible to 'mnemonic' these events by associating them with the facts you wish to learn.*
- Fill your thoughts with images and visions of yourself making the *exam* suffer for using up so much of your time. Aim for an elegantly detached matter-of-fact state in which there is just enough adrenaline and sympathetic activity to keep you alert and interested.
- According to Edison, genius is 1% inspiration and 99% perspiration. Many of your colleagues are saying that they have not done any work. What they really mean is that they have not done as much as they would like – and have actually done more than they realize, or are prepared to admit!

- This is a common phenomenon in the medical schools' game because the selection process seems to pick out many pathological perfectionists... they could *never* have done enough work and they rely on denial as a bizarre motivational strategy.
- This is fine because different people work in different ways. Your task is to recognize this and accept it. Nobody knows as much as you think they do – and you know more than you realize!
- Remember – nobody knows everything. Walter Mondale said, 'If you think you understand everything that is going on, you are hopelessly confused.' Make your learning efficient and ecological, and pay particular attention to your learning environment (see above).

Go for it

What you can do, or dream you can... begin it
Boldness has genius, power and magic in it

Goethe

Make it so!
Captain Jean-Luc Picard
(in *Star Trek: The Next Generation*)

People wish to learn to swim and at the same time to keep one foot on the ground

Marcel Proust

Goodness

To the good, be good
To the bad, be good too
In order to make them good as well
The He Zhizhang, Tang Dynasty

If you cannot speak good, be silent
Reported by Bukhari

The good is the beautiful
Lysis (Plato)

Internet

The Internet is a huge resource of study tips, notes, mnemonics and other people's PowerPoint™ presentations (ppts). Just beware of the validity of this information and also the fact that it may be out of date, or just plain wrong. Double-check and cross-reference the material unless you are very sure. See also the **Websites** listed below.

Key facts

You are aware of the concept of key words and key facts or phrases – to put it simply, those facts that will give you marks in the exam. Once you have gained an understanding of a topic, don't spend time learning anything unless it can be classed as directly relevant to obtaining exam marks. Once exams and assessments are no longer an issue, you can, of course, learn as many irrelevant facts as you wish! And have a good laugh about it. Even better, laugh all the way through your revision, too.

Laughter

When the first baby laughed for the first time, the laugh broke into a thousand pieces and they all went skipping about, and that was the beginning of fairies

Peter Pan

Maps and territories

The map is not the territory

Alfred Korzybski

Mind maps

Use mind maps or similar. These are surprisingly underused. Many of you will have come across them at school. Mind maps are especially useful for previewing a topic at the start of a study session, reviewing it at the end, and for making essay and project plans. I recommend any books or articles by Mind Map pioneer Tony Buzan if you would like to know more.

Mind maps are very useful if you are doing an exam with lots of sections or written parts. You start off by making several mind maps, one for each section. Then you start writing your answers. As you write, the earlier questions serve as memory joggers, and ideas will come for the later parts. You can immediately jot these down on to your other mind maps.

If you attempt to answer a question you think you know nothing about, doodling with a mind map can extract some answers from the inner recesses of your unconscious mind! Here's how to do one:

- Starting in the centre, write your topic or subject. Use plenty of colours and icons, images and doodles all the way through your mind map.
- Collect your key words and add them to the map.
- Connect each key word with a line to the central idea and also to other related areas of the map.
- Use thinner lines as you get further away from the centre.
- Use your own style.
- Remember, other people's mind maps tend to be less useful than the ones you created yourself.

The morning before the exam

Okay, so you're up, ideally having had a few hours of sleep to let yesterday's revision sink into your longish-term memory. Now have breakfast – unless, of course, you have done all of your learning on an empty stomach – see **Environment** above!

If you used caffeine during your revision, then have one cup of whatever you used, now. Skim through your cards, summarized notes, mind maps and mnemonics. Reinforce the material you have previously covered.

It makes sense to have at least an hour of mental relaxation just before the exam to let everything sink in and assimilate, allowing your neurotransmitter levels to recharge. You will need them at their peak to blitz these exams.

The night before

Get a few hours of quality sleep the night before – the rare exception to this rule is when you only have a single exam to do and really have done no preparation whatsoever. Having worked efficiently with plenty of breaks (see **Breaks** and **Environment**), you should be tired enough to get to sleep. The day/night before is usually when your mnemonics are most helpful (that is why we have made this book a portable size).

If you have a string of several days of exams, simply staying up night after night will turn you into a zomboid amnesiac, staring blankly at your exam paper.

While you sleep, your mind keeps working, sorting and assimilating what you have learnt. If you stay awake all night, learning lots of last-minute minutiae, you will certainly remember what you have just read in the last two hours or so (short-term memory) but are likely to have forgotten much of the earlier stuff. You decide if the trade-off is worth it.

Patients and preparation

The best preparation for tomorrow is to do today's work superbly well

To study medicine without reading textbooks is like going to sea without charts, but to study without dealing with patients is not to go to sea at all
Sir William Osler (1849–1919)
the most outstanding medical educator of his time

The secret of patient care is caring for patients
Peabody

Patterns

Students have used patterned representations for years to learn particular syndromes, for example for hypothyroidism, acromegaly, respiratory failure (pink puffers and blue bloaters) and so on. This includes photographs of rare patients with 'classical' signs, caricatures, drawings and – best of all – your personal memories of particular case studies. Medicine is, after all, much to do with 'pattern matching' and it will help during revision and self-testing also (although remember these are at best generalizations and their main purpose is to get you through tomorrow's exam).

Post-mortem (of exams)

The usual advice is to avoid these totally, but we all know that that doesn't happen in the real world. The best thing to do after an exam is to reflect a little then move on a lot.

Some students jot down what was asked, to prime their friends (or themselves for resits). I am told there are agencies which even pay you for this information.

Principle of precession

According to the 'principle of precession' by Buckminster Fuller, we gain many things on the way, in addition to the actual goal itself. The important thing may not be reaching the goal but how much we learn as we go along the way. The journey is as important in many ways as the piece of paper you are getting at the end.

The mirror reflects all objects without being sullied
The heart of the wise, like a mirror, should reflect all objects without being sullied by any

Confucius

Confucius did not probably intend a mirror to be a revision aid, but you can write on it with washable ink or stick on a Post-it™ note – one fact per mirror – which you never think about again, but as you look at the mirror each day it will become indelibly etched into your long-term memory (passive learning).

Problems?

Nothing lasts forever – not even your troubles!
Arnold Glasgow

... the problem is not the problem; the problem is the way people cope. This is what destroys people, not the problem. Then when we learn to cope differently, we deal with the problems differently – and they become different
Virginia Satir

... the package deal in being human involves problems, and it means we get to love to laugh to cry to try to get up and fall down and to get up again
Andrew Matthews

The way I see it, if you want the rainbow, you gotta put up with the rain
Dolly Parton

The mud puddles of life are only there to remind you it's just been raining
Stan Lee

Obstacles are things a person sees when he takes his eyes off his goal
E. Joseph Cossman

It is no good crying over spilt milk because all the forces of the Universe were bent on spilling it
William Somerset Maugham

If opportunity doesn't knock, build a door
Milton Berle

Record cards and Post-it® notes

Post-it® notes are handy for learning complex topics by breaking them down into smaller parts. One advantage is that the Post-its® can be arranged in different ways over books, notes, walls, bathroom mirrors, doors and wallpaper, for example.

Don't have more than one or two facts per note. Keep it simple. Avoid visual indigestion. Likewise, only have two or three notes per mirror or door (or posters, even). A whole wall with dozens of sticky notes on is an inefficient and time-consuming re-hashing process, although it may impress your flatmates! Within reason of course, you can do whatever you like. You can use the same sticky notes later, as bookmarks in different textbooks – which allows you to passively review the diagram or fact even while you are studying a completely different topic! Neat, huh!

Record cards can be used in a similar way.

Time is limited – once you've got it down on the cards/Post-it®, avoid duplication (yawn) of the same material. Instead, maximize remembering those facts on your cards by any means necessary. You can use your revision aids while walking or waiting for the bus, or in the dentist's waiting room. Their convenience lies in their portability. Remember that one or two clear bold facts, diagrams or mind maps per card is enough.

Regular breaks

We know that it is more efficient to study in sessions of 20–40 minutes and take regular breaks (e.g. 10–20 minutes). Yep, we talked about breaks earlier!

As well as keeping up your energy levels, and giving you a chance to share ideas and mnemonics with your friends, breaks allow you to *review* the stuff you just learnt and *overview* the stuff you are going to learn. Do this at the beginnings and ends of your study sessions.

Many people find that they get their best ideas and brain waves when they are most relaxed (e.g. in the shower, loo, bed). When you relax, you go into an alpha-wave state where you are at your most creative.

We have the best results in our life when we are prepared to go with the flow. This means finding the delicate and elusive balance between effort and relaxation, between attachment and letting go... Relax and let go – go with the flow

Andrew Matthews

Review, review, review!

Reviewing is the fundamental ingredient of all revision strategies.

So how does one review? Any way you like, although a few useful ways are to spend a few minutes (no more!) doing one of these things:

- Scribble down a mind map (2 minutes).
- Visually scan over the material in your mind's eye.
- Flick through your Post-it® notes or record cards.
- You can even go through your textbook or notes again (provided you only look *quickly* at the facts you have highlighted or underlined).

So when should you review? Ideally:

- At the start of your session (do a quick mental 2-minute overview of what you know of the topic – even if you think you don't know anything; it is permissible to look at past papers/previous years' tasks instead).
- After every paragraph or every few key facts (if paragraphs are irrelevant).
- At the end of the session (do a quick 2-minute visual fast-forward in your mind, like scanning on a video).
- After 24 hours.
- After 1 week.
- After 1 month.
- Pre-exam (this is usually the only time anybody else does it!)

Reviewing like this takes effort and seems to slow you down – but all this reviewing doesn't mean you need to spend hours slogging through lots of facts. Once you have gone through the material initially, you only need to review your key words, facts and phrases.

Reward

The highest reward for a person's toil is not what they get for it, but what they become by it

John Ruskin

Small is beautiful!

- Small *is* beautiful in the world of MBBS revision – get the smallest book on the topic. You always have lots of other information sources available, e.g. tutorials, handouts, friends, Internet, etc.
- Only use the minimal number of books per topic – a standard text, a crammer and a revision Q&A-type book is probably too much (but I will forgive you).
- Study groups can delegate workload to different students – you then teach each other. This is a terrific way to cover large amounts of material in a short time.

Smart drugs (nootropics or 'cognitive enhancers')

See Chapter 19, Nootropics.

Smile similes

Smile – it'll increase your face value

Smile and the whole world will smile with you

Smile – it'll squeeze out endorphins from those reluctant neurons

'Coz you smile when you feel good
And you feel good
When you smile

Various contributors

Staggering sessions

This does not refer to what you do on your way back from the medical school bar!

Staggering sessions means alternating your subjects. Study at least two topics at one sitting and make sure these are as dissimilar as possible. So, for instance, study anatomy for an hour or so, then alternate it with sociology and then biochemistry, before going back to anatomy.

You'll keep your mental energy levels up this way, while covering the same volume of material – and you'll retain more. This is because you'll avoid the fatigue associated with boredom. It gives those crucial neurons in the relevant section of your brain an hour's rest before returning to the original topic – as we know, different memories and different subjects use different sections of the brain. It is thus useful to know a variety of study methods.

Sticky wicket?

The man who removes a mountain begins by carrying away small stones
Chinese proverb

Commonsense is genius dressed in its working clothes
Emerson

Success is more attitude than aptitude
Johann Wolfgang Von Goethe

Failure lies not in falling down but in not getting up
Traditional Chinese proverb

Life can only be understood backwards; but it must be lived forwards
Soren Kierkegaard

Experience is the name everyone gives to their mistakes
Oscar Wilde

Study methods

Use any combination of study methods and keep them flexible!

Studying (like medicine) is really more of an art than a science. There are no absolutes! Be as flexible as you like... *as long as you take regular breaks and review often*, really any study method will work.

Suggestions include Tony Buzan's 'organic' method. This has defined stages including overview, preview, in-view, review, etc. This means that each topic is covered several times, looking at different aspects and different levels of detail each time. Other versions include the SQ3R – survey, question, read, recite and revise.

The secret is to find the most appropriate method for you, for that topic, for that time, and for that place – *as long as you take regular breaks and review often.*

Summarize

It has been said that you know you have learnt a topic if you can condense a huge wodge of notes down to the size of a postage stamp! A lot of the words are there to help you understand or they represent a writer's personal view of the Universe. Once you understand the material, let the low-value words evaporate and keep the crystallized mark-earning key facts, i.e. what you need to help you gain *marks.*

In practice, being able to chunk down a subject into a few pages or cards suggests that you understand the material. Then you only need to memorize the key facts. These key facts can be put on to a mind map for at-a-glance overview and review.

Effective summarizing explains the popularity of finals revision courses which condense the whole MBBS clinical course into a weekend – with good results.

So summarize. Summarize your summary, then summarize that. Then teach it to your colleagues and let them return the favour on another topic you don't have time for.

Taking yourself too seriously?

It is *only* an exam!

Keep things in perspective. If you want to exaggerate vivid thoughts in your mind, make sure they are thoughts about nice things in the world around you, all the positive things that have happened and will happen. Or of fabulous mnemonics! And even if you are really convinced you are going to have to resit your exam, revise anyway, because you will still need to know the stuff.

But, if you are really desperate to be serious about anything, be serious about humour!

But it does move

Galileo

Texts are tools!

Your texts are your servants – not the other way round! It is better to get your own books and **highlight**, <u>underline</u>, make notes in the margin, cross out waffly paragraphs, and whittle the words down to what is useful *now* to *you*.

Doing all this will help you learn because it uses visual, motor and auditory (say it to yourself, use mp3s, use music...) memory banks, all firing simultaneously. This is called neurological recruitment, and it works.

Remember, the text is your slave!

We get taught a lot of things that are never useful
Richard Bandler

Websites – some useful resources

Almost a Doctor: www.almostadoctor.co.uk

Ask Doctor Clarke: www.askdoctorclarke.com

BMJ Best Practice: www.bestpractice.bmj.com

Breaking Bad News: www.breakingbadnews.co.uk

Dr Najeeb Lectures on YouTube: www.youtube.com

Khan Academy revision notes: https://www.khanacademy.org/science/health-and-medicine

OSCEstop: www.oscestop.com

Medic 2 Medic: www.medictomedic.org.uk

PasTet: www.pastest.co.uk

United States Medical Licensing Examination (USMLE) video tutorials and first aid book: www.usmle.org

Will Weston revision: http://westonnorth.co.uk/revisionnotes/index.html

Wisdom and knowledge

One of the greatest pieces of economic wisdom is to know what you do not know
John Kenneth Galbraith

Can your learned head take leaven
From the wisdom of your heart?
Lao Tse (translated by Witter Bynner)

And finally...

They know enough who know how to learn
Henry Adams

Enjoy!

INDEX